CANCER

Herbs in Holistic Healthcare

by Dr J. Walker

Published by
Amberwood Publishing Ltd
Rochester, England

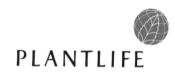

PLANTLIFE

Registered Charity No. 328576

Amberwood Publishing supports the Plantlife Charity,
Britain's only charity exclusively dedicated to saving wild plants.

ISBN 1-899308-28-8

Cover design by Studio Read

Printed in Great Britain

CONTENTS

About the Author

Dr Walker trained as a Doctor of Medicine and Doctor of Surgery at the University of Sheffield and qualified in 1977. Initially she worked as a Physician and Surgeon in local hospitals and later, after further training, moved into General Practice where she was a Principal for over 15 years, during this time she had a special interest in gynaecology and HRT. She also had a part-time commitment at a local hospital as a Casualty Officer and later as a Genito Urinary Physician.

Since leaving the NHS in 1995, she has expanded her knowledge of medical hypnotherapy, acupuncture and herbal medicine as a complimentary adjunct to conventional medicine and has studied at The School of Phytotherapy in East Sussex.

Dr Walker has had several articles published about plant based medicines, in *Update*, a journal of continuing medical education for general practitioners and in *The European Journal of Medicine*.

She married Colin in 1976 and has one son, Robert; her hobbies include gardening, music, lace making, crotchet and embroidery.

Note to Reader

Whilst the author has made every effort to ensure that the contents of this book are accurate in every particular, it is not intended to be regarded as a substitute for professional medical advice under treatment. Readers are urged to give careful consideration to any difficulties which they may be experiencing with their own health and to consult their General Practitioner if uncertain as to its cause or nature. Neither the author nor the publisher can accept any legal responsibility for any health problem which results from use of the self-help methods described.

Acknowledgements

This book is the culmination of many years of medical practice and I am indebted to so many people for their comments and support. Most of all I would like to acknowledge my many patients particularly those who have been kind enough to give me constructive feedback and criticisms on various treatments.

Thanks must also go to my immediate family who have given unwavering emotional support both when things have gone well and when they haven't; for discussing ideas on presentation and for their attempts to curb my medical jargon and make the book more 'readable'.

Thanks also to June Crisp and her supportive team at Amberwood.

There are hundreds of problems and hundreds of herbal remedies, I've discussed some of them with many people particularly local Members of the Institute of Medical Herbalists and taken their suggestions and supportive comments on board. Thanks also to Dr John Cosh who was kind enough to read and comment on the book and has written the foreword and Andrew Chevallier, a herbalist of many years experience for his comments. I would also like to thank Dr Leonard Mervyn for his comments on the section about vitamins and minerals and for his time taken in writing to me with correct values.

It seems also appropriate to acknowledge my medical teachers at the University of Sheffield who taught me the value of thorough clinical examination and the application of logic in making the correct diagnosis. Thanks must also go to my teachers at the School of Herbal Medicine in Bodle Street Green in East Sussex particularly the late Hein Zeylstra for opening the world of Herbal Medicine up to me.

Foreword

Cancer in its various forms can give rise to a wide range of unpleasant symptoms, either due to the disease itself, or its treatment, or to the fear associated with it. In this book we read of the drugs commonly used in the conventional treatment of cancer, and of their many possible side effects.

From her many years of experience, the author is able to advise on herbal remedies, which can be used instead of conventional drugs, alleviating symptoms effectively and safely.

This information is backed up by sound advice on a holistic approach to health care. The guidance given here will be of value both to cancer sufferers and to their families.

Dr John Cosh MD FRCP

Preface

Life is short, the art long, opportunity fleeting, experience treacherous, judgement difficult. The physician must be ready, not only to do his duty himself, but also to secure the co-operation of the patients, of the attendants and of externals.

Hippocrates (c460BC–357BC) APHORISMS I

I have been a doctor for 25 years, and believe that the task of all physicians is to help the sick, in whatever ways we can. Various tools are available to us including many medications, synthetic and natural.

This book aims to inform patients, their doctors, nurses and other health care professionals about safe, effective, natural remedies that can be used to treat some of the unwanted effects or concurrent illnesses associated with cancer and its treatment. They may also help to improve mental and physical health following chemotherapy or radiotherapy.

Four out of ten people will develop cancer at some time in their lives. In the UK approximately 220,000 people will be newly diagnosed each year, so chances are high that you, or someone close to you, will suffer from cancer. The reason more of us are being diagnosed with cancer is because we are living longer.

The good news is that statistics show that more people than ever are surviving cancer because of great strides in research and the development of new regimes to treat the disease. Many of these regimes utilise medicines derived from plants. Professor Gordon McVie, Director of the Cancer Research Campaign said, "We are on the eve of a revolution which will see a whole range of new, effective treatments. Cancer may not be cured by the year 2050 but it will be beaten and the disease will be as readily controlled as diabetes is today."

This is not intended to be a book about the herbal treatment of cancers, as there is little research into the role that many of the plant medicines could play in this, except in the laboratory. At present I believe there is no herbal magic bullet just as there is no universally effective drug regime for cancer. However, botanical (herbal) medicines have been shown to play a part in the management of cancer and in many health problems that may occur at the same time.

I also believe that patients should seek thorough investigation and treatment from an oncologist (cancer specialist) whose results are in line with international predicted cure/survival rates.

I have practised independently from the NHS for a number of years, during which time herbal and nutritional solutions figured largely in my regimen for helping patients. I am still disappointed to find that some family and hospital doctors remain sceptical about the benefits of natural medicines, when patients tell me how well they feel when taking them.

In this book I have included herbs with a long history of traditional use where I consider that this acts as their clinical trials. Often these herbs are prescribed for similar health problems in the herbal pharmacopoeiae of several different countries.

We now understand the solid scientific basis for these treatments. In the 1970s research confirmed the specific antibiotic, diuretic or anti-inflammatory effects of some herbs claimed by herbalists for generations and this research continues.

More recently new drugs have been synthesised entirely in the laboratory and pharmaceutical companies are eager to get them on the market to recoup their investment as soon as possible.

Researchers from Toronto found that adverse drug reactions kill more than 100,000 people in the USA per year which makes legitimately prescribed medicines the fourth biggest killer there, behind heart disease, cancer and strokes. I believe that, because of other similarities in the way we practice medicine here in the UK, the proportions per head of population are similar, so we may be looking at up to 40,000 deaths per annum from prescribed medications.

In the UK, Charles Medawar, of the drugs-monitoring group *Social Audit* said that up to five per cent of all hospital admissions were due to reactions to prescribed drugs and drugs that have been bought over the counter. Once in hospital 15 per cent of in-patients have their treatment affected by a drug reaction, 50 per cent of which, the group says, could be avoided.

In my experience herbs are extremely safe when administered correctly. I rarely see adverse reactions to a plant-based medicine and if they occur, these tend to be minor and self-limiting, resolving completely when the herb is discontinued.

On the other hand, manufactured drugs commonly cause unwanted effects that adversely affect our health.

At present we do not know how many people experience unwanted effects from drugs but it undoubtedly amounts to tens of thousands of patients per year. Some reports of adverse reactions are not taken seriously because doctors know of no link between the unwanted symptoms and the active ingredient contained in the medication.

All drugs contain a number of inert ingredients as well as the pharmaceutical product. Some 700 or so other chemical agents are used as additives to make them look and taste appealing and to prolong shelf life. Some colourants are known to cause hypersensitivity reactions, including dermatitis, asthma, urticaria and rhinitis. There is now increasing evidence that additives can produce unwanted effects. For example aspartame which is used as a sugar substitute in liquid medicines, especially those intended for children and the elderly, are known excitotoxins which can precipitate headache, seizures and panic attacks.

Some effects are not considered serious or significant enough to merit either hospital admission or a 'yellow card' report to the Medicines and Healthcare Products Regulatory Agency. Indeed, the fatigue caused by beta-blockers is so commonplace that most family doctors simply accept its occurrence as inevitable, even 'normal'. When the unwanted effect is a problem like depression or insomnia, lifestyle problems are usually blamed rather than the prescribed drug.

Potentially fatal bleeding from the gut caused by non-steroidal anti-inflammatory drugs (NSAIDs) such as Diclofenac, prescribed for arthritis, gout, and back pain affects thousands of patients per year, many of them in older age groups where health is generally more fragile.

I don't believe that herbal preparations can completely replace synthetic drugs. But natural and synthetic substances can complement each other, with those who care for the health of others being aware of the advantages and the shortcomings of both.

This appears to be the situation in many European countries where physicians and pharmacists prescribe plant medicines in conjunction with orthodox medicine. In France, only qualified medical practitioners are allowed to prescribe herbal medicines and the majority do utilise them. In Germany, pharmacists dispense herbal medicines which are, like drugs, licensed for certain illnesses. In the UK many herbal products can be purchased as food supplements from delicatessens and health food shops as well as pharmacies. Because they are considered to be 'food' they are not subjected to the same scrutiny as drugs. Now we are in the European Community it seems probable that this will be reviewed.

About this book

My primary aim is to provide guidance and advice to people who have been diagnosed with cancer, or who have a friend or relative with cancer, who wish to take alternative or herbal remedies for concurrent health problems safely, with or instead of pharmaceutical products. However, you don't have to suffer from cancer in order to benefit from these natural remedies.

Each chapter deals with a particular problem such as anxiety, depression or insomnia. I have tried to deal with the types of drugs that you might be prescribed first and include possible unwanted effects experienced by other patients who have taken them.

Sometimes, statistics are included to show the percentage of patients who have experienced a specific unwanted effect when taking a drug compared to those who have suffered that effect when taking a placebo. This should illustrate how likely it is that you might suffer a particular unwanted effect. I have also included a few statistics comparing the effectiveness of a herbal treatment against a pharmaceutical product widely used for the same sort of problem.

I also include suggestions for lifestyle and dietary changes and conclude each section with details of beneficial herbs. Some of these herbs have been proven to help by clinical studies (usually in Europe or the USA), while others have a long history of traditional use in these particular problem areas.

Main reference works are included. The full list of references is on my web-site at www.aaron-associates.com in the publications section.

In the section on each herb are its main uses for a particular illness, unwanted effects (if any), interactions with other herbs or drugs, and any reasons why the herb should not be taken at all. I have included all reports of unwanted effects that I have been able to find, even if the link with the herb was not proven.

Many herbs are not recommended during pregnancy and while breastfeeding because there is no research available to confirm their safety.

Recommended dosages of herbs are included and the many ways that herbs can be prepared. Generally, herbs are taken by mouth three times daily, either as a tablet or capsule, an infusion (tea), decoction (strong solution in water), tincture (preparation of the herb in alcohol or glycerol to aid preservation), liquid extract or fresh herb juice. Fresh herb juices are generally pasteurised, when prepared commercially, to extend their shelf life. You can, of course, prepare your own with a juicer.

Injecting herbal extracts into the body is not recommended because, although the plant chemicals in them are safe if taken into the body through the gastro-intestinal tract, if injected, they may have unwanted effects. The most likely adverse reaction is haemolysis (breakdown of the red blood cells) because of the high levels of steroidal saponins.

Many herbs can be taken as a tablet or capsule, which I recommend for the herb that you use as your main medication. You may prefer to take liquid extracts, fresh herb juices or tinctures. You can safely use more than one herb at a time. Refer to the interactions sections to avoid possible problems.

Sometimes adding another herb as an infusion (tea) or decoction several times a day will increase the action of the main herb, or you may wish to combine one or more herbs as a tincture or liquid.

Some patients prefer to use glycerol instead of alcoholic tinctures, including people with primary or secondary liver cancers and recovering alcoholics. Some drugs, such as Metronidazole (Flagyl), are contraindicated when taken with alcohol since the drug blocks its natural breakdown in the liver. This causes elevation of unwanted chemicals in the body and leads to feelings of nausea and general malaise. It is unlikely to cause health problems in the doses used in herbal medicines but patients may prefer to avoid any possible conflicts in their treatments.

The usual dosage is based on an average of 70kg of body weight. For people over 65 years of age best results are obtained by commencing treatment at the lower end of the dosage scale and working upwards as required.

Keep to recommended doses for your particular problem Usually, these are taken from *The British Herbal Pharmacopoeia* (1983). Many people think that herbs are perfectly safe and dosage is not an important issue. However, I believe that it is not possible to think of herbs as effective therapeutic agents without also believing that, if taken in overdose, they could have undesirable effects. Many years of use along with meticulous observation has gone into calculating the safe medicinal dosage of herbs. This is now often backed up by modern research findings, so be grateful to these past and present herbalists and use their knowledge wisely.

If you can make a cup of tea you can make a herbal infusion. The only difference is that you must cover the infusion and leave it for at least 10 minutes to brew. Capsules and tinctures can be easily purchased from reputable sources.

Note that there may be other interactions, either adverse or beneficial, of which we are unaware.

1 | Anxiety

Before the cherry orchard was sold everybody was worried and upset, but as soon as it was all settled finally and once for all, everybody calmed down, and felt quite cheerful. ~ Anton Chekhov (1860-1904) *The Cherry Orchard*

For centuries herbalists have used single herbs or a combination of herbs to relieve symptoms of anxiety.

Anxiety is a normal human response to uncertainty, which drives us to make changes that are productive and useful. For example, students who are anxious about their exams will study more and are more likely to be successful.

However, when a situation is not in our direct control we cannot respond in the same active way to our anxiety. It therefore remains and brings about changes within the body that are unhealthy.

It is normal for people who have cancer to feel anxious about their illness and concerned and uncertain about their future and that of their family. For many of you this is just a natural phase of your illness, driving you to seek medical advice and make decisions about your treatment. Usually, once a diagnosis has been made and a treatment strategy has been decided and embarked upon, most people feel calmer and more in control of their lives and illness. However, some of you will continue to feel anxious and this may cause upsetting symptoms.

In some people anxiety just causes a feeling of tension, but in others troublesome and distressing physical symptoms may also occur. These can fall into the following categories:

Increased tension in muscles leading to:
- Tiredness
- Trembling
- Restlessness and sleeplessness

- Muscle tension, such as tension in the neck muscles that can give rise to persistent headaches.

Overactivity of the autonomic (automatic) nervous system resulting in:

- Shortness of breath
- Rapid heartbeat
- Dry mouth
- Cold hands
- Dizziness

Increased vigilance leading to:

- A feeling of being 'keyed up' or 'on edge'
- Increased jumpiness
- Impaired concentration

Relatives and friends may also suffer from acute anxiety symptoms. Sometimes they continue to feel anxious because it is not always possible or feasible for them to take a direct part in treatment decisions.

Often support, advice and reassurance are all that are required, but sometimes, because of persistent or troublesome symptoms, you may seek medical help. You might be prescribed medication that includes one or more of the following drugs:

A. Anxiolytic drugs (technically called hypnotics, sedatives and tranquillisers). Usually benzodiazepines such as oxazepam or diazepam are prescribed for the duration of your treatment. These drugs bind to specific receptor sites in the brain, prompting it to produce anxiety-reducing chemicals. They should never be taken for more than four weeks at a time.

In 1989, 21 million prescriptions for hypnotics, sedatives and tranquillisers were issued by the NHS (the vast majority for benzodiazepines) at a cost of some £34m (£27m for benzodiazepines). However, in general the trend is falling. It is estimated that some 1.5 million people are addicted to this group of drugs, although there are no accurate figures available. Some 50 per cent of patients admitted to hospital in the early 1990s became tranquilliser addicts as a result of a brief hospital admission.

B. Antidepressants. Some of these – for example Imipramine, Prozac, Seroxat, Venflaxine and Paroxetine – are as effective as benzodiazepines in some people with anxiety symptoms.

C. Some doctors prescribe stronger drugs that have an effect on brain chemistry. They are actually antipsychotic drugs. Trifluoperazine has been found to reduce anxiety but has many more side effects than most other drugs.

D. Sometimes other drugs such as beta-blockers are used because, although they have different side effects, they cause less sedation. All beta-blocker names finish with the suffix -olol, for instance atenolol, propranolol. They have not been adequately evaluated for use in anxiety but are widely prescribed.

E. Busipirone may be prescribed because it is effective in anxiety states, though its beneficial effects take longer to become apparent than with benzodiazepines.

F. Hydroxyzine is marketed for use in patients with anxiety. However, research involving 1344 patients found no significant reduction in anxiety with this product.

G. Abecarnil is also used for patients with anxiety. Research showed no benefit over placebo in clinical trials.

H. Barbiturates are rarely used nowadays because of the number of side effects and high risk of addiction.

Unfortunately, many of these drugs can lead to short-term and long-term side effects. You may find that having successfully addressed the problems of your cancer treatment, you now have new problems secondary to the treatments given to help to relieve your anxiety.

A. The benzodiazepine group of drugs are known to cause the following unwanted effects:

- Most of these drugs have a depressing effect on brain chemistry and consequently on the whole body. Tranquillisers are also known to damage brain receptors and cause neurotransmitter imbalance. This is now recognised as a major factor in developing addiction. Patients who take benzodiazepines feel low, slow, sedated, light-headed, drowsy (71 per cent v 13 per cent with placebo) and depressed. The drugs also slow down mental agility, impair attention span, reasoning, short-term memory and concentration making daily living more difficult and adding to your difficulties as a cancer patient.

- An increased risk of Parkinson's disease.

- Reaction time is slowed so patients taking this class of drug should always be advised not to drive a motor vehicle or operate machinery.

- Many people experience something known as potentiation, where the body becomes accustomed to the standard dose, and they need to take ever-increasing amounts to achieve the same effect.

- Many patients feel numb, unable to respond to the normal ups and downs of life – known as emotional blunting. There may be increased dependency on friends, relatives or medical staff, as the patient is unable to make everyday decisions about life. Ability to make an informed judgement about treatment may be impaired and there may be memory loss and impairment from the time the drugs are taken until they are excreted from the body some hours later. Some patients exhibit inappropriate behaviour while taking these drugs, in particular an increase in mood swings and even uncharacteristically aggressive behaviour.

- Benzodiazepines have a variety of effects on sleep pattern – they alter rapid eye movement sleep or very deep sleep (REM sleep). This alteration of sleep pattern may take months or even years to return to normal so many people feel that they cannot sleep when they stop taking benzodiazepines. This can be apparent even if the drugs are not being used as a sleeping pill. If the drugs are suddenly stopped, disorientation, insomnia and even hallucinations can occur.

- Excessive salivation, gastric irritation, nausea and constipation have been reported.

- Other effects are numerous and range from impotence to incontinence. Some types of benzodiazepines can also lead to an increased risk of falls in the elderly. Falling can be a major hazard, especially for older people and those who already suffer from other physical disabilities where it can lead to hip fractures and other serious health problems.

- Benzodiazepines can affect normal function of the thyroid gland.

- Research has shown a 17-fold increase in fatal heart attacks in patients taking this class of drug.

- Biochemical effects of benzodiazepines within the body lead to dependency even after a short period of use. This is because of alterations in body chemistry, and unpleasant physical and mental symptoms will usually occur if the drugs are suddenly stopped. These include headache, muscle pains, extreme anxiety, tension, restlessness, confusion and irritability.

- Many patients suffer from withdrawal symptoms. They describe problems that occur on stopping the drug to be worse than the original problem(s) for which they were prescribed. Withdrawal symptoms from tranquillisers can persist for well over 10 years in a substantial proportion of patients. Benzodiazepine addiction can lead to brain atrophy.

- It is possible to stop treatment with this group of drugs but this must be carried out under professional supervision.

- Benzodiazepines have adverse effects in pregnancy. Babies born to women who took benzodiazepines during pregnancy have brain and nerve damage and develop neuro-behavioural problems. Research by Dr James Robertson of Liverpool's Arrowe Park Hospital showed that one in two babies exposed to benzodiazepines in pregnancy ended up in intensive care. This compared to one in seven babies exposed to hard drugs such as heroin. A survey by a Tranx charity showed that nine out of ten children born to women who took benzodiazepines during pregnancy have an Attention Deficit Disorder and/or personality problems. This compares to only one in 10 in the general population. They have also been found to be more susceptible to developing other ailments such as epilepsy, ME, mental illnesses, panic attacks, eye problems, facial developmental problems, renal abnormalities and heart defects.

- Benzodiazepines can affect other medicines. It is inevitable that a patient undergoing chemotherapy or radiotherapy will take other drugs at some time during their course of treatment.

- Some other drugs increase the effects of benzodiazepines – oral contraceptives, hormone replacement therapy, anaesthetic agents, Isoniazid, Cimetidine, Omeprazole, Fluvoxamine, Fluoxetine, alcohol, other sedatives including herbal sedatives, and sedative antihistamines such as Chlorpheniramine.

- Some other drugs decrease the effects of benzodiazepines – they include antacids, tobacco, Rifampicin, and Cisapride.

- Research has shown conflicting results but it is reasonable to conclude that the use of benzodiazepines at the same time as anti-epileptic drugs makes side effects and toxicity more evident.

B. Antidepressant drugs are known to cause the unwanted effects described on page 42.

C. Trifluoperazine is known to cause the following:

- Over-stimulation including increased anxiety and agitation. There are records of patients becoming dependent on Trifluaperazine.

- Unusual involuntary muscle movements have been noted occasionally but are unusual when patients take a normal dosage. Trifluaperazine may also induce symptomatic Parkinsonism.

- An irregular or rapid heartbeat may occur. Some patients have had problems with low blood pressure leading to falls and fainting. This may be postural, that is it may occur on standing from a sitting or lying position. Other patients have noticed different effects on the cardiovascular system including chest pains.

- Nausea and vomiting are commonly experienced.

- Inflammation of nerves in the feet and hands may occur, also difficulty in passing urine. Some patients taking this drug have had episodes of sweating and pallor sometimes followed by flushing. Sensitivity to light is an occasional side effect.

- Rare instances of blood abnormalities and abnormal bruising have occurred.

- Trifluoperazine interacts with a large number of other medicines such as anti-depressants, benzodiazepines, some cold cures and also some common foods such as Marmite, Bovril, red wine and other alcoholic drinks, mature cheese, pickled foods such as onions and gherkins, and broad bean pods (these contain levadopa).

D. Surveys of patients show that about 25 per cent of patients who take beta-blocker drugs experience adverse effects. They are known to cause the following:

- Beta-blockers can lower the blood pressure and may cause a sudden drop in blood pressure when standing from a sitting or lying position. This can cause unsteadiness and result in fainting and/or falls. They may also reduce the pulse rate to unacceptable levels, making patients feel faint. Many people on these drugs feel tired and lacking in energy. Ability to exercise may be reduced.

- Cold extremities, making conditions like Raynaud's syndrome worse.

- Depression. Because of the circumstances for which beta-blockers were prescribed it is often not recognised as an unwanted effect of the medication and is thought to be a natural progression of the patient's anxiety state. In addition, confusion, dizziness, headache, mood changes, nightmares and sleep disturbance have all been experienced. Serious psychiatric disorders have occasionally been linked to these drugs.

- Worsening of any symptoms due to diabetes, heart failure and angina leading to difficulties in controlling these illnesses, whether they are pre-existing or develop throughout the period of treatment for cancer.

- Dry mouth, indigestion, anorexia, acute pancreatitis, jaundice, abdominal pain and cramps, diarrhoea and constipation. Occasionally beta-blockers have been thought to cause liver damage.

- There have been recorded cases of thrombocytopenia (low platelet count) and abnormal bruising.

- Disorders of the skin, hair and eyes, which include dry eyes, hair loss, a skin rash resembling psoriasis, worsening of existing psoriasis and other allergic-type skin rashes.

- Muscle/leg cramps and generalised aching in joints.

- There have been several recorded cases of visual disturbance.

- Beta-blockers will almost certainly make existing asthma worse and may bring on latent asthma causing shortness of breath and wheezing.

- Difficulty getting an erection – this is a common side effect and is caused by changes in the circulation to the extremities. Some women also experience sexual difficulties. This can lead to increased feelings of anxiety in either sexual partner.

- Researchers have noticed that older male patients treated for high blood pressure with beta-blockers have twice the incidence of cancer as control patients.

- Memory problems have been demonstrated in patients taking beta-blockers.

- More serious reaction to a variety of allergens if taken by someone with a history of allergy. They may also reduce the response to adrenaline, often given in emergency treatment for acute allergy.

E. Buspirone is known to cause the following:

- Effects on brain function. It is less likely to cause significant sedation than benzodiazepines but some patients taking Buspirone feel dizzy (64 per cent v 12 per cent on placebo), sleepy (19 per cent v 7 per cent on placebo) light-headed, and nervous. Headache can also occur. No evidence of dependency has been found.

- Different effects on the cardiovascular system. These include rapid pulse, palpitations and chest pains.

- Significant numbers of patients experience nausea (34 per cent v 13 per cent on placebo).

- Other effects such as sweating, dry mouth, tiredness, and confusion have occasionally been reported.

F. Hydroxyzine is known to cause the following:

- Drowsiness is the most common unwanted effect (10 per cent).

- Headaches are also frequently experienced (6 per cent).

- Dry mouth may occur.

- Dizziness, weakness and confusion.

- Rarely tremor and unwanted movements may occur. Convulsions are very rare.

G. Abecarnil is known to cause the following:

- Drowsiness (47 per cent).
- Dizziness (16 per cent).
- Irritability (9 per cent).
- Unsteadiness (5 per cent).
- Decreased libido (5 per cent).

These safe, alternative non-drug strategies are proven to help ease anxiety:

Counselling

It often helps to discuss your fears with a counsellor, GP, your consultant or nurse. If you have a specific worry he/she may be able to reassure you.

A study in 1998 concluded that 50 per cent of GP practices offered counselling. Reassuringly 99 per cent of counsellors had relevant qualifications and appropriate levels of clinical supervision. Usually appointments with a counsellor last longer than with your GP, which will give you time to discuss your feelings and worries. He/she may also be qualified to use cognitive therapy – this is a term used to describe therapy that is a mixture between relaxation training, systemic desensitisation and cognitive behavioural therapies, found to be superior to relaxation alone. There were no unwanted effects in response to this type of treatment.

Stimulants

Avoid stimulants such as coffee, cola drinks, chocolate, strong tea and herbs intended to give more energy, which usually contain *Cola nitida*, *Ephedra sinensis* or *Paullina cupana* (guarana). These all contain the psychoactive substance caffeine, and may cause a dramatic increase in feelings of anxiety and even trigger panic attacks.

Many people find substituting bottled or filtered water or non-stimulating herbal teas such as linden or chamomile (see later) very helpful. Decaffeinated tea and coffee may be acceptable, but some people react badly to the chemicals used in decaffeination.

Sugar
Try to reduce your sugar intake. Cutting down on sugar, sweets, cakes and biscuits can improve mood and reduce anxiety symptoms.

Alcohol
Reduce or avoid alcoholic drinks – alcohol has a tendency to increase current emotions. It may also trigger panic attacks.

Diet
Improve your diet and nutrition. When you are unwell your appetite may decrease and food intake becomes erratic and ill balanced. Deficiencies of certain minerals and vitamins have all been linked with anxiety. These include the B vitamins, vitamins C and E, calcium, magnesium, phosphorus, potassium, selenium, omega-3 and omega-6 essential fatty acids. If stress is long term your requirement for these vitamins may increase. You may wish to take supplements if your appetite is poor. Your GP, practice nurse or Macmillan nurse should be able to advise you.

Try to include complex carbohydrates such as wholemeal bread and cereals, potatoes and other vegetables, wholemeal and root vegetable-based pasta, in your diet. Eat a little at every meal if you can – they have a natural tranquillising effect.

In a recent large-scale South African study it was found that a daily multivitamin tablet was more effective than a placebo in reducing anxiety.

Sweeteners
Take special care to avoid artificial sweeteners such as aspartame (E951). These are found in many products, such as snack foods, diet drinks, yoghurts, fruit squash, and vitamin supplements, so read the labels carefully. Aspartame can alter the production of natural mood regulating hormones in the brain, increasing feelings of anxiety. Large amounts have caused panic attacks.

Aromatherapy
Soothing oils such as lavender, sandalwood, jasmine and melissa can have a calming effect. Try blending oils that you feel comfortable with. Use five to ten drops in an oil burner, added to your bath water or dripped onto your pillow at night. A weekly aromatherapy massage from a registered masseuse can have a relaxing and anxiety-reducing effect. It will leave you

with a sense of well-being by helping to relax muscles that tend to tighten up when you feel anxious.

Exercise
Exercise stimulates the brain to produce natural anxiety-reducing chemicals. Any physical activity can be effective although you may wish to check with your health practitioner before embarking on a new or more strenuous activity. Recreations like bowls or dancing are not only physically beneficial but add an enjoyably positive social aspect to your life.

Breathing
If you are anxious you may hyperventilate or 'overbreathe'. When this happens your breathing becomes too shallow and rapid, resulting in light-headedness and dizziness and increased feelings of anxiety. Concentrating on breathing slowly and deeply will help you to relax.

Relaxation
Meditation and relaxation have a powerful effect on the body. Research has shown that they boost immunity, and relieve insomnia and other anxiety-related symptoms. Relaxation tapes can be helpful or your GP may refer you to a support group or counsellor.

Hypnosis
Some GPs and counsellors offer hypnosis as a way of coping with anxiety and I have found this very effective for a large number of patients. Self-hypnosis (auto-hypnosis) can be very helpful as an aid to relaxation if practised regularly. It can also prepare you to relax for events such as receiving anaesthetic for an operation, a minor operation under local anaesthesia or administration of intravenous chemotherapy.

Humour
Your sense of humour is a powerful ally in your quest for healing and has been proven to reduce anxiety and improve mood. A good laugh triggers the release of endorphins – chemicals in the brain that produce feelings of euphoria and relaxation. Production of cortisone is also suppressed – this is the hormone produced in excess by the body when it is under stress. Too much cortisone can lead to a rapid pulse and high blood pressure.

Emergency relief

Here are some quick tips for rapid anxiety relief. Researchers have found that anxiety feelings intensify when we look down. Try to concentrate on looking upwards or scan the horizon – either will help symptoms to abate. At the same time lower your shoulders to release muscle tension in your neck region.

You may also notice that your speech becomes more rapid and that the pitch of your voice rises when you are anxious. Make a conscious effort to slow your speech and lower the pitch of your voice. Try to combine this with deeper, slower breathing to help you feel calmer and convey a feeling of calm and control to others. This is especially useful when meeting a new specialist, preparing for treatment or when you are in any situation that you find stressful.

If symptoms continue or are very troublesome there are effective, safe and non-addictive herbal alternatives to conventional tranquillisers.

Valerian ~ *Valeriana officinalis*

Valerian root has been used for centuries to calm anxiety and relax muscles. It has been thoroughly researched and its effects have been confirmed as a tranquilliser, antispasmodic and mild analgesic.

In a remarkable series of experiments it has been found to be sedative, useful for anxiety states including panic attacks, palpitations and sweating. Unlike drugs used for the same problems, it can actually improve co-ordination.

Central nervous system sedation is regulated in the brain by GABA-A receptors. It is thought that the constituents of valerian bind to these sites and therefore exert a calming effect.

A vast amount of research has been carried out into valerian. While it produces a feeling of calmness, it does not affect wakefulness or alertness. It even helped to prevent the sedating effects of alcohol and actually increased concentration and energy levels. Valerian is very useful in calming nervous excitability and stress, providing a useful alternative to the benzodiazepines.

It does not appear to affect the ability to drive, nor operate machinery, nor does it significantly increase the effects of alcohol or result in a morning hangover.

There is no risk of dependence and tolerance.

For years low doses of valerian have been prescribed to ease the pain of muscle spasm and cramps. Valerian increases the effect of painkillers either herbal or drug-based so it is useful to take where painkillers are not fully effective and tension and anxiety are present.

It also helps to lower blood pressure where anxiety is a causative factor.

Higher doses promote restful sleep – see chapter 3.

Valerian is quite safe. In an attempted suicide a patient took 40-50 x 470mg tablets, which resulted in only minor side effects – tiredness, abdominal cramps and a feeling of being light-headed – from which the patient made a full recovery.

Uses
- Acute and chronic anxiety
- As a muscle relaxant
- To increase the effects of painkillers
- To aid withdrawal effects in patients addicted to benzodiazepines
- Pre-menstrual tension
- Migraine headaches
- Insomnia
- Leg cramps

Unwanted effects
- Sometimes slight headache, giddiness
- Rare allergic reactions
- Occasional restlessness, usually if larger doses are taken

Interactions with other herbs
- Increases the effect of other sedative herbs
- Increases the effect of other painkilling herbs

Interactions with drugs

- Barbiturates
- Sedatives, such as sleeping pills or benzodiazepines
- Alcohol
- Anaesthetic agents

Contraindications

- Imminent general anaesthesia
- Liver disease

Recommended dosage
All three times daily

Tablets/capsules	200mg
Fresh herb juice	10ml
Dried rhizome and root	0.3-1g
Liquid extract (BPC 1963) 1:1 in 60% alcohol	0.3-1ml
Tincture Simple (BPC 1949) 1:8 in 60% alcohol	4-8ml
Concentrated infusion (BPC 1963) 1:5 in 25% alcohol	2-4ml

Chamomile flowers ~ *Matricaria recutita*

German chamomile flowers are frequently used to reduce anxiety. This herb is suitable for all age groups and is one of the most well-known and researched medicinal plants in Europe. It is a much milder herb than valerian and is useful for daytime relaxation, having a general calming effect. The flowers are the effective part – taking the whole plant is not recommended.

There are two distinct plants known as chamomile:

A. Roman Chamomile (*Chamaelirium nobile*), previously known as *Anthemis nobile*.

B. German Chamomile (*Chamomilla recutita*), previously known as *Matricaria chamomilla*.

Although they are both called chamomile, the chemical composition of the two plants is not the same. Roman chamomile is slightly bitter, and less strong than German chamomile, which is generally more anti-inflammatory and pain relieving. Because of this I favour Roman chamomile for children whilst German chamomile is the herb of choice for most adults.

German chamomile has clear anxiety-reducing effects in normal doses (in the region of 30mg/kg), without demonstrating muscle-relaxing, sedating or anticonvulsant activity. At doses between 30-100mg/kg, mild sedation is produced.

Research shows that its antispasmodic effects are comparable to the drug papaverine. One of the natural component chemicals of chamomile, apigenin, was found to be more than three times as active. Apigenin is also anti-inflammatory.

The natural chemicals that give chamomile flowers their yellow colour, the flavones (*flavus* = Latin for yellow), are active in the central nervous system, lowering anxiety levels. Chamomile yields a blue essential oil that can be utilised either in skin care or diluted with a carrier oil and massaged into the skin as a relaxant.

Chamomile tea is readily available in most supermarkets or health food stores. The best results are obtained from dried flowers – shop-bought tea bags can give poor results. It is a very useful substitute for tea and coffee as it does not contain caffeine. Some people may find chamomile and spearmint or one of the other chamomile/herb combinations have a more acceptable flavour.

Uses
- Anxiolytic (anxiety-reducing)
- Sedative
- Treatment of gastro-intestinal spasm and irritation

Unwanted effects
- Rare anaphylactic reactions
- Contact with the fresh plant or the tea may cause contact dermatitis or allergic conjunctivitis in sensitive individuals.

Interactions with other herbs
- Increases the effect of other sedative herbs

Interactions with drugs
- Warfarin and other anticoagulants
- Benzodiazepines and other sedative drugs
- Alcohol

Contraindications
- Pregnancy (whole plant – a tea made of flowers only is acceptable in small amounts)
- Sensitivity to the plant or other plants in the *asteracea* family such as chrysanthemum
- Existing use of anticoagulants

Recommended dosage

Dried flower heads	6-24g or by infusion daily
Liquid extract 1:1 in 45% alcohol	3-12ml daily
Tincture	3-12ml daily
Essential oil on a sugar lump	6-9 drops daily

Motherwort ~ *Leonurus cardiaca*

Motherwort can be used as a sedative. Its action is similar to valerian, and it is very good for treating panic attacks and palpitations with its generally calming effect on the heart. As its common name implies, it has a special affinity for women and is helpful for patients who suffer from anxiety, irritability and mood changes, especially during the menopause. It has antispasmodic and sedative actions, aids relaxation but does not cause sleepiness.

Research in China shows that this herb relaxes heart cells, and may help to prevent the blood clots that trigger heart attack. Some research in animals has shown improvement in coronary circulation mainly by slowing the heart rate and increasing the efficiency of contraction.

Preliminary research findings in Russia have suggested that the herb contains natural substances that lower blood pressure.

Uses

- Panic attacks, especially if accompanied with palpitations
- Anxiety
- Antispasmodic

Unwanted effects

- A theoretical risk of photosensitivity

Interactions with other herbs

- Increases the effect of other sedative herbs
- *Digitalis purpurea* (foxglove)

Interactions with drugs

- Theoretical risk of some interaction with Digoxin but this has never been demonstrated
- Anti-coagulants such as Warfarin and other drugs that inhibit blood clotting.
- May increase the effect of other sedative drugs and beta-blockers

Contraindications

- Pregnancy
- During heavy menstrual bleeding
- Blood-clotting disorders

Recommended dosage

Dried herb or by infusion	3-12g daily
Liquid extract 1:1 in 25% alcohol	6-24ml daily
Tincture 1:5 in 45% alcohol	6-36ml daily

Linden (or lime flower) ~ *Tilia europea*

The flowers or complete flower heads and bracts of the lime or linden tree make a pleasant tea or infusion that is mildly tranquillising and sedative. It helps to calm those who are over-excited or unduly anxious, relieving nervous tension. The herb is widely believed to combat high blood pressure. It is widely used on the Continent as an after dinner tisane/infusion known as *tilleul*.

Linden also appears to improve digestion and acts as a general calming agent on the gastro-intestinal tract, so it is especially useful when anxiety is combined with loss of appetite, colic or digestive upset.

It is widely believed to combat the build up of fatty deposits in the blood vessels that may lead to the development of arteriosclerosis but I have been unable to find any studies to confirm this.

Uses

- Anxiety
- Stress
- Nervous tension
- Colic
- Diarrhoea, flatulence and heartburn

Unwanted effects

- None

Interactions with other herbs

- None

Interactions with drugs

- None

Contraindications

- None

Recommended dosage

Dried flower heads with bract by infusion	6-12g daily
Liquid extract 1:1 in 25% alcohol	6-12ml daily
Tincture 1:5 in 45% alcohol	3-6ml daily

Passionflower ~ *Passiflora incarnata*

Spanish explorers first discovered this plant in the Peruvian Andes in the middle of the 16th century. The Incas had used it medicinally for hundreds of years.

There are several hundred plants in the *passiflora* family. Some have similar sedative properties to *Passiflora incarnata*, but others are either not pharmacologically active or contain undesirable chemicals. As most data has resulted from research into *P incarnata*, I recommend that you use this variety, which is the one found in proprietary teas and tablets.

The plant's name comes from its beautiful and unusual flowers, seen to signify Christ's Passion. Its main action is, in fact, not likely to induce passion as it is mildly sedative and tranquillising. It also has marked anti-spasmodic properties, confirmed by researchers. Passionflower's effects are particularly useful where anxiety and tension are present and where getting to sleep is a problem (see chapter 3).

In animal experiments it has been found to lower blood pressure, stimulate respiration and to act as an analgesic.

Passionflower has traditionally been used as a painkiller for tension headaches and other minor pains. It may help to increase the effects of stronger painkillers.

Experimental studies have shown that some of the substances in passionflower dilate the coronary arteries so it may be useful in heart conditions.

It is non-addictive.

Uses

- Anxiety
- Stress
- Insomnia

Unwanted effects

- May cause drowsiness in higher doses

Interactions with other herbs

- Will increase the effect of other sedative herbs

Interactions with drugs

- May occur with MAO inhibiting antidepressant drugs.
- May increase the effect of other sedative drugs

Contraindications

- Pregnancy and breastfeeding

Recommended dosage

Dried herb by infusion	1.5-7.5g daily
Liquid extract 1:1 in 25% alcohol	1.5-3ml daily
Tincture 1:8 in 45% alcohol	1.5-6ml daily

English Lavender ~ *Lavandula angustifolia*

Almost everyone is familiar with the lovely fragrance of lavender and it is well known for its gentle sedative effects. It relieves both anxiety and depression and there can be few people who aren't aware of the benefits of a few drops of essential oil of lavender as an aid to relaxation in the bath, sprinkled onto the pillowcase, or used in an oil-burner. It can be diluted with vegetable oil for massage or taken internally.

Oil of lavender is used for massage in many hospices for its overall relaxing action. It can alleviate mild pain, enhance the effects of other painkillers and relax restless patients.

Lavender can be taken internally to treat restlessness and mood disturbance, also for abdominal cramps and menstrual discomfort. It has been used externally in conventional medicine as a massage oil for rheumatic diseases and headache.

Modern research confirms its sedative properties. Researchers have shown that lavender increases the effects of other sedatives and analgesics.

In another study subjects who inhaled lavender oil showed sedation, and relaxation responses. Unlike the drug Nitrazepam, it had no effect on heart rate or reaction time.

Lavender has a low toxicity but significant antibacterial action and is useful for treating the very young and very old.

Uses

- Irritability and restlessness
- Insomnia or poor sleep
- Headache and migraine
- As a disinfectant

Unwanted effects

- None

Interactions with other herbs

- Increases the effect of other sedative herbs

Interactions with drugs

- May increase the effect of other sedative drugs

Contraindications

- Pregnancy

Recommended dosage

Dried flowers by infusion	3-6 g
Essential oil of lavender BPC (1973) on a sugar cube	1 to 2 drops (0.06-0.12ml)
Tincture 1:5 in 60% alcohol	6-12ml daily
Compound lavender tincture BPC (1949)	6-12ml daily

2 | Depression

The only sure foundations of medicine are, an intimate knowledge of the human body, and observation on the effects of medicinal substances on that.

~ Thomas Jefferson (1743-1826)

Depression is an illness that makes you feel miserable over a long period of time. There may also be physical changes such as weight loss. It is caused by chemical changes within the body and brain that lead to abnormal feelings.

Unfortunately, many people who feel depressed are told to 'pull themselves together' or 'cheer up' by well-meaning friends and relatives and even sometimes by their medical attendants. Most people who are experiencing a depressive illness would love to do this but unfortunately it is rather like telling someone who is experiencing a heart attack to relax. Chemical changes within the body are completely out of control.

People who are depressed have difficulty coping with everyday life and in making choices. It remains the most common psychiatric problem among adults. Around six people per 100 will experience a depressive illness at any one time in the UK, and one in three people will suffer a depressive illness at some time in their life. Some people seem to be more susceptible to depression than others. This includes patients who have long-term physical illnesses. Women are twice as likely to become depressed as men and you are more likely to feel this way if you have experienced a depressive illness in the past.

Stressful situations or other illnesses can bring about these changes in the body. Some drugs used in the treatment of cancer can lead to depression. It may also occur after a general anaesthetic or childbirth.

Many patients experience feelings of helplessness, despair and self-blame after being told that they have cancer. In addition, surgery, chemotherapy and radiotherapy can lead to malaise, weakness and other physical symptoms which trigger the sort of chemical changes that can lead to a depressive illness.

It must be stressed that depression can be a serious illness, and if you think that you are suffering from it you should seek professional help from your health practitioner as soon as possible.

Depression is an eminently treatable condition and responds well to herbal medicines if mild to moderate in severity. Severe depression may require hospitalisation and will certainly need stronger psychotropic drugs, rather than herbs, to bring it under control. If neglected, depression can lead to worsening of your symptoms, feelings of despair, an inability to function normally and, occasionally, to suicide.

If you develop a depressive illness you may notice some or all of the following symptoms:

- A persistent low mood and general loss of interest in things that you normally find interesting.
- Feelings of worthlessness, hopelessness, despair or of guilt, often over inconsequential issues.
- Difficulty sleeping, often with early morning waking although sometimes excessive sleeping may be a symptom.
- Difficulty making decisions.
- Many patients lose the ability to experience pleasure.
- Decreased energy and lack of motivation.
- Feelings of agitation or restlessness.
- Lack of concentration and forgetfulness sometimes occur.
- Your appetite could be decreased and weight loss usually occurs; sometimes you may feel like overeating, usually a particular food such as chocolate or ice cream.
- Increased alcohol intake may be a feature of depression because some patients drink to try to escape from unpleasant feelings.
- Some people experience physical symptoms such as aches and pains or headaches.
- You may have crying episodes for no apparent reason.
- Some people have decreased sexual interest, ability and enjoyment.

- A few patients have suicidal ideas and/or thoughts of death.
- Delusions and/or hallucinations are rare but may be a feature of your illness.

Depression can also be a symptom of other medical conditions such as:

- Hypothyroidism or myxoedema (an inadequately functioning thyroid gland).
- Anaemia (low red blood count, usually because of insufficient iron or sometimes vitamin B12 or folic acid).
- Menopause (see chapter 13).
- Liver disease including liver tumours, both primary and secondary.
- Kidney disease.
- Brain tumours, including secondary cancer.
- Senility and dementia.

Some medicines are known to cause depression.

If you are taking any of the following medicines do **not** stop them yourself but discuss them with your doctor who should be able to suggest an alternative.

- Painkillers such as codeine.
- ACE Inhibitors, such as Enalopril, used for hypertension.
- Vasodilators – used in heart disease.
- Anti-epileptic drugs such as Carbamazepine.
- Steroids such as Kenalog (Triamcinolone) or Prednisolone.
- Beta-blockers such as Atenolol, or Propranolol (see page 22).
- Methyldopa – used for hypertension.
- Statins – used for lowering cholesterol.
- Oral contraceptives, in some women.
- Hormone Replacement Therapy, in some women (see page 160).
- Diazepam and other benzodiazepines (see page 18).
- Sleeping pills such as Flunitrazepam (see chapter 3).
- Barbiturates.

- Reserpine.

- Anti-arrhythmics.

- Anti-Parkinsonism drugs.

- H2 antagonists such as Ranitidine and Cimetidine (see page 92).

- Amphetamines.

- Anti-arthritic drugs/NSAIs such as Diclofenac.

- Recreational drugs such as cannabis and Ecstasy.

Sometimes, as in the case of anxiety when a diagnosis of cancer has been confirmed, investigations have been completed and treatment has commenced, you will begin to see things in a more positive light and to feel better without any specific treatment at all.

Many GPs and specialists tend automatically to write a prescription for one of the frequently prescribed 31 or so antidepressant drugs on the market.

There are four main groups of antidepressant drugs:

- Tricyclic anti-depressants.

- New tricyclic and related antidepressants.

- Selective antidepressants such as SSRIs (Selective serotonin reuptake inhibitors).

- Monoamine oxidase inhibitors known as MAOIs and reversible inhibitors of monoamine oxidase.

There is plenty of evidence that side effects are very common and usually affect at least five per cent of patients overall. Thirty per cent of patients treated with tricyclic anti-depressants stopped taking them because of unwanted effects. Patients taking SSRIs didn't fare much better, with 27 per cent of patients stopping treatment because of unwanted effects. In a series of post mortem examinations from 1979-1989, tricyclic antidepressants were found to be a causal factor in 12 per cent of deaths.

From 1958-1977 nearly 600 deaths of children under 10 years were attributable to accidental poisoning by drugs, usually tragically mistaken for sweets. After 1970 tricyclic antidepressants were the most common drug implicated in accidental poisonings in this age group.

Unwanted effects of antidepressant drugs include:

- Uncharacteristic feelings of agitation, anxiety and nervousness which may be accompanied by insomnia. Occasionally patients develop feelings of aggression. Some patients feel apart from reality – so-called depersonalisation.
- Dizziness and low blood pressure, which can lead to a fall. In older patients and those with other health problems this may increase the tendency to fractures and risk of further illness.
- Headache (10-15 per cent) is a frequent unwanted effect. It usually subsides when treatment is stopped.
- Dry mouth (10-15 per cent), loss of appetite, diarrhoea, nausea, constipation and occasionally gastro-intestinal bleeding has occurred.
- Excessive sweating.
- Feelings of drowsiness, fatigue, malaise, tiredness and sedation.
- Tremors can occur. Some types of antidepressant such as Flupenthixol are known to induce symptoms of Parkinsonism.
- Visual problems, such as blurred vision – this may improve even if the drug is continued.
- Loss of libido and other sexual difficulties in as many as 75 per cent of patients taking SSRIs.

Other regularly reported, but less frequent (1-5 per cent) side effects include:

- Difficulty passing urine.
- Loss of concentration.
- Confusion and hallucinations.
- Halitosis (bad breath).
- Nightmares and vivid dreams.
- Loss of memory.
- Withdrawal symptoms on trying to stop treatment. These have included dizziness, sweating, tremor and confusion. Such symptoms have often been so bad that they resulted in the reinstatement of the drug, despite claims from drug companies that they are 'safe and easy to discontinue'.

- Abnormal liver function tests.

- Increased suicidal tendencies in patients who take Fluoxetine (Prozac).

In addition to these, some rarer unwanted effects have been reported:

- Patients were 2·4 times more likely to suffer hip fracture than those not taking the drug. SSRI antidepressants were the most dangerous but other types also carried increased risk.

- One of the most concerning is low blood sodium associated with inappropriate secretion of ADH.

- Patients taking tricyclic antidepressants may have decreased vitamin B levels.

- Women who have taken some types of antidepressants in pregnancy are more than twice as likely to give birth to babies with physical abnormalities.

- It has been claimed that modern anti-depressants are safe in overdose (either deliberate or accidental). However, evidence is accumulating that this is not so, and there have been reports of heart abnormalities, coma, sweating and hyperventilation and seizures in patients taking more than the normal dose. Several patients have died.

It should be noted that side effects are more common in patients over 60 years of age.

Special precautions are needed in some patients with the following conditions:

- Epilepsy.

- Diabetes mellitus.

- Patients with blood disorders affecting blood clotting.

- Abnormal heart rhythms.

In June 1992 the Citizen's Commission on Human Rights in the USA said: 'More than 23,067 adverse reactions by Prozac users have been reported to the Food & Drug Administration (in the USA) since Prozac's release in 1987 (including 1436 suicide attempts and 1313 deaths). These include delirium, hallucinations, violent hostility and aggression, psychosis and attempted suicide. Major medical journals have reported the emergence of suicidal thoughts in persons taking Prozac.

CANCER: HERBS IN HOLISTIC HEALTHCARE

'In the last year, nearly 50 lawsuits have been filed against Eli Lilly seeking almost one billion dollars in damages by families of people who have committed suicide while on Prozac, families of people who have been murdered by patients on Prozac, and people who have been themselves damaged while taking Prozac'.

Disturbingly, there are several accounts of people exhibiting atypical violent, even murderous behaviour, while taking these drugs.

There are now firms of lawyers in the USA who specialise in taking on the drug companies for patients who claim to have been harmed by taking these legal, legitimately prescribed antidepressants. I have no reason to think that this will not occur here in the UK.

These lifestyle changes will help if you feel depressed

Counselling

Sharing your feelings and other worries with a counsellor, GP, consultant, practice nurse, Macmillan nurse or a close friend or family member may be helpful. If your GP practice has the facility you may be offered a consultation with a psychotherapist/counsellor. These are professionals who are specially trained to help you to discuss problems such as depression. A review of depressed patients treated either by their GP or a counsellor demonstrated higher levels of satisfaction when they were seen by the counsellor.

Psychotherapy

Since some level of depression in people who have cancer is perfectly understandable, referral to a psychiatrist would be inappropriate because they are trained in the treatment of abnormal mental processes.

However, if you have a long history of depression or recurrent depression you will almost certainly benefit from seeing a psychotherapist. Depression can be the result of many factors, stressors and situations associated with everyday life and the development of your illness. Several non-drug treatment strategies are effective in treating chronic and/or recurrent depression including hypnosis.

Diet

When depressed, most appetites are reduced, and this includes desire for food. However, you do need to pay special attention to your diet. Make sure that it is well balanced and contains fresh fruit and vegetables daily. Avoid junk food, supermarket ready meals and so-called cook-chill foods, as they tend to be high in salt and low in essential vitamins and fibre.

Eat some wholegrain foods every day such as brown rice, lentils, barley or wholemeal bread. Also ensure that there are sufficient essential fatty acids in your diet such as fish oil, oil of evening primrose, linseed oil, hemp seed oil, olive and other mono-unsaturated oils. A relative lack of these fats has been implicated in a range of psychiatric conditions including depression. They can also be found in sunflower seeds, pecan nuts, pumpkin seeds and nuts in general.

Hot spicy food, including cayenne pepper and other hot spices, produce endorphins that improve mood.

If your appetite is poor, it is good idea to take appropriate supplements until you feel better. Your health practitioner can advise otherwise take a good general multi-vitamin and mineral supplement. Researchers at the University of Calgary treated patients with calcium, iron, copper, selenium and other minerals – results were good with patients able to come off medication and return to work.

Take B vitamins, particularly vitamin B6, folic acid, thiamine, riboflavin and vitamin B12. Lowered levels of these vitamins have been linked to depression.

Caffeine

Cut out caffeine – it is a psychoactive drug of great power. When we are depressed we tend to drink more caffeine-containing drinks such as tea, coffee, chocolate and cola but they can make us feel worse. Chocolate sweets and bars are also a source of caffeine.

Smoking

Avoid smoking cigarettes and taking mood-altering drugs. They may give a short term 'high' but are not helpful in the long-term.

Aspartame

Avoid foods and drink containing aspartame. This artificial sweetener has been shown to decrease natural antidepressant chemicals in the brain. More seriously, in a clinical study, when depressed patients were given aspartame, they exhibited such bizarre and worrying behaviour that the study had to be abandoned. Unfortunately, aspartame can also be found in some vitamin supplements from a well-known chain of chemists, so you need to read labels carefully.

Alcohol

Cut out alcohol. It makes depression worse and may lead to dependency problems. Many people with cancer tend to drink alcohol to escape from unwanted or unpleasant feelings. Alcohol can also cause depression but not necessarily. It tends to be a mood enhancer. If you feel a little down in the dumps then drinking alcohol will tend to make you feel worse.

Alcohol can also impair transport of the amino acid tryptophan to the brain. Normally, tryptophan is converted to serotonin, a natural mood-regulating chemical. In addition to this, long term regular alcohol consumption can lead to shortage of vitamin B especially if your appetite is also impaired.

Exercise

Exercise has been proved to stimulate your levels of brain hormones and makes you more alert and motivated. German researchers studied the effect of exercise on 12 patients, the majority of whom had failed to respond to drug treatment – all the patients improved. In more than 50 per cent the improvement in mood was substantial. There were no adverse effects and no one quitted the study. Even a short walk daily will improve circulation and encourage production of beneficial hormones.

Light therapy

Some people become depressed in the winter months when daylight hours are diminished, and sunlight levels are lower even on a bright day. It is thought that a certain intensity of sunlight is necessary to stimulate a hormone called melatonin. When melatonin levels fall, depression can follow. Sufferers can benefit from high intensity light therapy. Your GP should be able to advise you further.

Relaxation

Learn how to relax using relaxation exercises, tapes or music. Yoga, meditation or massage all help to relieve tension, anxiety and irritability caused by depression. Your GP should be able to advise you and may refer you to a support group or counsellor.

Bibliotherapy
Research has shown that written material or audio tapes helped some people to combat depression but that they probably only suffered a mild form. Your GP, Macmillan nurse or even your local library should be able to provide suitable materials.

Befriending
In a small study of 86 patients, 65 per cent were helped by meeting someone socially, once a week for one hour. This will be most useful for people who don't have a large circle of friends. There are often local support groups for those who are coping with cancer and its treatments. Your Macmillan nurse should be able to advise you. Often there are support groups for relatives too.

Rest
Slow down your pace of life and don't be afraid to take regular breaks during the day. This is especially important if you are having treatment such as radiotherapy.

Keep occupied
A hobby, reading a book or even watching a good film on television will prevent you from dwelling on your depression and help you feel better. Be selective about what you view on TV. Regularly watching some programmes especially soap operas and others with depressing storylines can adversely affect mood.

If your symptoms continue or are very troublesome, there are a number of herbal remedies that are effective, safe and non–addictive.

St John's Wort ~ *Hypericum perforatum*

St John's wort has a long history of medical use. It was described by Hippocrates and Plinius in ancient times and by Paracelsus in the Middle Ages. The aerial parts of the plant are used medicinally. It is only comparatively recently that St John's wort has been found useful in treating depression.

In a randomised, double blind, parallel group trial, published in September 2000 in the *British Medical Journal*, St John's wort was found to be equivalent to Imipramine in treating mild to moderate depression; but patients tolerated St John's wort better (St John's wort 39 per cent v Imipramine 63 per cent).

There are at least 27 studies involving over 1800 patients showing that St John's wort is as effective as most of the antidepressants used for mild to moderate depression.

In a recent analysis of 23 randomised trials of mild to moderate depression involving 1757 patients, it was concluded that St John's wort was significantly superior to placebo and probably as effective as drug treatment but with fewer side effects (19.9 per cent v 52.8 per cent on antidepressants).

In eight trials (1123 patients), which compared St John's wort to other antidepressant tablets, the herb was associated with significant clinical improvement compared to placebo but not with standard antidepressants. However, compared to the antidepressants, patients taking St John's wort experienced fewer side effects. Other reviews came to the same conclusions.

In a randomised, double blind trial lasting six weeks involving 149 outpatients, St John's wort was compared to Fluoxetine (Prozac). Researchers concluded that 800mg of St John's wort daily was equivalent to 20mg Fluoxetine.

In an Austrian study, 67 per cent of patients with mild to moderate depression improved when given St John's wort.

Like drug treatments, the herb's full effect is not evident for four to six weeks. In my opinion because it has fewer side effects patients feel better while taking it and are therefore more likely to continue treatment, and resolve their symptoms.

Some patients with more severe illness will not benefit from St John's wort. If the recommended doses (see later) do not help your symptoms don't be tempted to take more. There is no evidence that doses above the normal range are any more effective and they may result in a higher incidence of side effects.

St John's wort is the most commonly prescribed antidepressant in Germany and is widely used in other European countries. It is not currently licensed as an antidepressant in the UK so preparations will claim to be the 'sunshine herb' rather than a proven antidepressant remedy.

Uses

- Mild to moderate depression
- Fatigue
- Menopausal problems

Unwanted effects

- Photodermatitis – unlikely in normal therapeutic doses.
- Increased sensitivity to touch, temperature and pain in four cases, all were taking high doses of high potency preparations.
- Fatigue.
- Dizziness.
- Pruritis.
- Weight gain.
- Mood changes and emotional vulnerability.
- Gastrointestinal symptoms such as nausea, constipation, and abdominal discomfort.
- Possible cataract formation.
- Allergic reaction.
- Headache.
- Dry mouth.
- Sweating.

Interactions with other herbs

- Will increase the effects of sedative herbs

Interactions with drugs

Many studies have found that St John's wort uses the same liver pathways for its metabolism as some commonly prescribed drugs and also some common foods such as cruciferous vegetables, ethanol (alcohol), and nicotine. It makes good sense therefore not to take the following drugs with St John's wort:

- Tricyclic antidepressants, such as Amitriptyline, Imipramine and Doxepin.

- Selective serotonin reuptake inhibitors (SSRIs) – antidepressants such as Fluoxetine, Sertraline and Paroxetine. This has resulted in the so-called serotonin syndrome, consisting of dizziness, nausea, headache, confusion, stomach pain, anxiety and confusion.

- Oral contraceptives containing oestrogen. Two pregnancies have been reported.

- Antibiotics such as tetracyclines and sulphonamides.

- Thiazide diuretics.

- Theophylline.

- HIV protease inhibitors such as Indinavir, Nelfinavir, Ritonavir, and Saquinavir.

- HIV non nucleoside reverse transcriptase inhibitors such as Delaviridine, Efavirenz, Nevirapine.

- Digoxin.

- Cyclosporin.

- Warfarin.

- Cimetidine.

- Triptans prescribed to relieve migraine – Sumatriptan, Naratriptan, Rizatriptan and Zolmitriptan. It has been suggested that hypericum and Triptans could interact.

- Anaesthetic agents.

- Reserpine.

- Sedatives.

- Iron – tannins in St John's wort may inhibit absorption.

- Sildanefil.

- Over-the-counter cold and flu preparations.

Contraindications

- Severe depression
- Imminent general anaesthesia
- Pregnancy

Recommended dosage

Products standardised to 0.3% hypericin are recommended.

Tablets 200-300mg	5-10 tabs daily (total 2-4g daily)
Fresh herb juice	30ml daily
Dried herb by infusion	2-4g daily
Liquid extract 1:1 in 25% alcohol	6-12 ml daily
Tincture 1:10 in 45% alcohol dose	6-12 ml daily

I recommend that St John's wort is taken for six weeks. If there is no improvement (although the full response may take up to three months), it should be stopped and a different therapy tried.

Skullcap ~ *Scutellaria laterifolia*

Skullcap has a long history of use in North America, although it is a relative newcomer to the European herbal repertoire. In the 1896 edition of the *National Formulary*, Stillé & Maisch indicated its usefulness 'in depressed and disordered conditions of the nervous function'. The aerial parts of the plant are used in remedies.

Skullcap is classed as a relaxing nervine and has many uses but is particularly helpful to patients with a long history of depression or those who have become depressed after a long illness or after surgery. Many herbalists believe that there is nothing better for the nerves than skullcap.

There are records of it being prescribed for patients with depression caused by illness, over-exertion and 'long continuing and exhausting labours'. It has also been used for pain, epilepsy and high blood pressure.

Uses
- Depression
- Sedative
- Antispasmodic

Unwanted effects
- Large doses are said to cause light-headedness

Interactions with other herbs
- Increases the effects of sedative herbs

Interactions with drugs
- Sedatives
- Immunosuppressants

Contraindications
- Pregnancy and breastfeeding

Recommended dosage

Capsules/tablets	3 x 200mg daily
Dried plant by infusion	2-6g daily
Liquid extract 1:1 in 25% alcohol	6-12ml daily
Tincture 1:5 in 45% alcohol	3-6ml daily

Lemon Balm ~ *Melissa officinalis*

This lemon-scented herb has been used for centuries to lift emotions in mild depression but it also calms anxiety, restlessness and irritability. It reduces feelings of panic and palpitations and has a secondary effect in calming the gut, relieving indigestion, over-acidity, nausea, bloating and colicky pains. Lemon balm also shows powerful viro-static properties. In Germany it is approved for use in nervous conditions.

If picking the herb from your garden pinch out the tender leaves at the tip for a more intense lemon flavour.

Uses
- Mild depression
- Anxiety states
- Stress
- Nausea secondary to emotional upset
- Hyperthyroidism

Unwanted effects
- Minor gastric upsets when used in high dosage

Interactions with other herbs
- Increases effects of other sedative herbs

Interactions with drugs
- Barbiturates and Primidone
- Thyroxine
- Sedatives

Contraindications
- Hypothyroidism
- Glaucoma – theoretical risk of increasing pressure in the eye
- Pregnancy and breastfeeding

Recommended dosage

Fresh herb, by infusion	6-12g daily
Fresh herb juice	30ml daily
Liquid extract 1:1 in 45% alcohol	6-12ml daily
Tincture 1:5 in 45% alcohol	6-18ml daily

Oats ~ *Avena sativa*

Oats are a popular and nutritious cereal, and there is little doubt that porridge made from them benefits health and lowers blood cholesterol levels. It is used as a medicinal plant all over the world. For medicinal purposes the whole plant is usually gathered when the grain is ripe.

Oats have been used for centuries to improve stamina and treat general debility and mild depression. Biochemical analysis reveals numerous natural chemicals known to be neuro-muscular stimulants, enhance repair of tissues and increase feelings of motivation and drive.

Some steroids in *Avena sativa* release more endogenous testosterone into the system, thus having a beneficial effect on sex drive and mood, motivation and general well-being. Avenin is a neuro-muscular stimulant that increases stamina and endurance.

In Ayurvedic medicine *Avena sativa* is prescribed to treat withdrawal from drugs such as nicotine and opium.

Oats are traditionally used to raise energy levels gently and support an over-stressed nervous system.

Uses

- Mild depression
- Stress
- Fatigue
- Convalescence

Unwanted effects

- None

Interactions with other herbs

- None

Interactions with drugs

- Morphine

Contraindications

- Coeliac disease

Recommended dosage

Avena sativa may need to be taken for at least a month for effects to be noticed but can be safely taken for long periods.

Fresh herb juice	30ml daily
Liquid extract 1:1 in 25% alcohol	1.8-6ml daily
Tincture 1:5 in 45% alcohol	5-10ml daily

Vervain ~ *Verbena officinalis*

Historically vervain was associated with witchcraft, sorcery and superstition and was largely employed as a panacea. More recently it has proved useful in treating post-operative depression and depression occurring after chemo- or radio-therapy.

Vervain is known to relieve tension and stress without causing drowsiness. It moderates autonomic nervous activity and has a relaxing, calming and restorative effect on the nervous system. It has a gentle action free of side effects and can benefit even the most debilitated patients.

This herb also has minor anti-inflammatory and analgesic properties. Research in Europe has identified a weak anti-oedema action.

The aerial parts of the plant are used in remedies.

Uses

- Depression
- Convalescence, particularly post-operative
- Stress-related problems such as headache

Unwanted effects

- None

Interactions with other herbs

- None

Interactions with drugs

- None

Contraindications

- Pregnancy
- Heart failure
- Asthma
- Colitis, and other chronic gastrointestinal complaints

Recommended dosage

Dried herb by infusion	6–12g daily
Liquid extract 1:1 in 25% alcohol	6–12ml daily
Tincture 1:1 in 40% alcohol	15–30ml daily

3 | Insomnia

The beginning of health is sleep ~ Irish proverb

Insomnia is a perception of insufficient or poor quality sleep.

Sleep seems to be a time of rest and relaxation, but it is really a period of great physiological activity with dramatic variations in hormonal secretion such as growth hormone (which peaks during sleep). Brain activity is altered with recurrent cycles of short brain waves and rapid eye movement.

As yet the function of sleep is not fully understood. It is known, however, that too little sleep leads to general fatigue, difficulties with memory, thinking processes and to depression.

When a patient receives a cancer diagnosis, it is normal for them to experience a period of sleeplessness and there is no need to prescribe medication, either drug or otherwise, unless it becomes prolonged or affects the quality of life during the day.

Insomnia can also be a symptom of other medical problems such as depression, anxiety, asthma or even prostate problems, which might cause nocturia (the need to get up in the night to pass urine). Pain may also lead to difficulty in sleeping and to relieve insomnia here, the important issue is to control the pain.

Many women notice a change in their sleep pattern at the menopause. Thirty per cent of adults experience insomnia during the year. It becomes more common with increasing age and women are twice as likely to be affected as men.

Often drugs prescribed to treat insomnia cause psychological or physical addiction, increasing the patient's health problems.

Some drugs can cause sleeplessness themselves; others may induce poor sleep by causing nightmares and other sleep disturbances. If you are taking any of the drugs listed below and experience difficulty in sleeping, contact

CANCER: HERBS IN HOLISTIC HEALTHCARE

the doctor who prescribed them. It may be possible to change them for another medication. Do *not* stop taking them without medical advice.

- Antidepressants such as Fluoxetine (page 42).

- Non steroidal anti-inflammatory drugs such as Ketoprofen can disturb sleep either by leading to agitation or by causing nightmares.

- Steroids by mouth such as Prednisolone.

- Selegiline, a treatment for Parkinson's disease.

- Thyroxine may cause insomnia; it is usually an indication of overdosage.

- Diuretics such as Frusemide and Bendrofluazide tend to produce more urine and stop the usual reduction in urinary volume at night time, thus waking you to pass water.

- Pseudoephedrine (ie Sudafed) can cause sleeplessness and hallucination.

- Cafergot suppositories can cause agitation and sleeplessness.

- Theophylline, such as Theo-Dur and Slo-Phyllin may cause restlessness and insomnia.

- Salbutamol, Terbutaline and Bambuterol, can lead to feelings of tension which interfere with sleep.

- Hydralazine can lead to agitation and insomnia.

- Amantadine.

- Some liquid preparations of drugs contain aspartame as a sweetener. This is a known excitotoxin and can produce sleeplessness. Formulations change from time to time so please consult your pharmacist or the product information enclosed with your medication for this information.

Drugs used for the treatment of insomnia

Hypnotics – these are usually benzodiazepines such as flunitrazepam. Nowadays, short-acting benzodiazepines are used to minimise the problem of daytime drowsiness and hangover such as Zalepon and Zolpiden. These should never be prescribed for more than one month because of the risk of dependency.

Antidepressants – some, such as amitryptiline, are prescribed to improve sleep.

Sedative antihistamines – such as chlorpheniramine and diphenhydramine, are available in over-the-counter preparations such as Nytol. Promethazine is sometimes prescribed to aid sleep. All these drugs interact with benzodiazepines, antidepressants and alcohol.

Chloral hydrate – this central nervous system depressant is sometimes prescribed. It interacts with benzodiazepines, antidepressants and alcohol.

These drugs are known to cause the following unwanted effects

Benzodiazepines – these are covered in detail on page 18.

Antidepressant drugs – these are described in detail on page 42.

Sedative antihistamines – are known to cause the following unwanted effects:

- Dizziness (6 per cent), drowsiness (4.5 per cent) and grogginess (7 per cent) are most frequently encountered.

- Loss of appetite can happen, gastric upset and constipation have occurred

- Rarely, tic-like movements, muscle spasms and uncontrollable limb movements have been noted.

- An increased risk of delirium has been identified in older patients, often associated with disorganised speech and mistaken for a stroke. Behavioural disturbance and bladder problems have occurred, requiring catheterisation.

- Dry mouth, blurred vision, nausea and nervousness have also been reported.

- Headaches, nightmares and disorientation occur rarely.

- These medicines may thicken lung secretions and impair coughing and should not be used in patients with lung diseases or breathing problems such as asthma, bronchiectasis, cystic fibrosis and bronchitis.

- They should be avoided in patients with raised pressure in the eye/glaucoma, peptic ulcer; coronary disease, epilepsy, liver or kidney diseases.

CANCER: HERBS IN HOLISTIC HEALTHCARE

- A low platelet count occurs occasionally.
- Some people experience sensitivity to light, giving rise to a skin rash on exposed skin.
- These drugs are not recommended in pregnancy and breastfeeding.

Chloral hydrate – is known to cause the following unwanted effects:
- Abdominal distension, gastric upset and bloating
- Damage to the tissue of the kidney.
- Headache sometimes occurs.
- Sweating, hot flushes and variable blood pressure including raised blood pressure.
- Delirium, especially in the elderly.
- Allergic skin rashes are rare.
- Not recommended in pregnancy and breastfeeding.
- It should not be prescribed for patients with porphyria, liver disease or those taking anti-coagulants,

Some drug-free ways to relieve insomnia
The bedroom is for sleep and sex only. If you watch television there or catch up on your letter writing or reading you will lose the psychological impetus for sleep.

Stimulants
Avoid stimulants of any kind. This includes ingested stimulants such as cola drinks, coffee, tea, chocolate and chocolate flavourings. The effects of caffeine can last for up to 20 hours so even a cup of coffee in the morning can lead to disturbed sleep! Illegal drugs such as Ecstasy and amphetamines are also stimulants, which may result in a disturbed sleep pattern. Some over-the-counter medicines may contain caffeine.

Stimulating herbs that excite should also be avoided, such as *Cola nitida, Paullina cupana* (guarana), and *Ephedra sinica.*

Other less obvious forms of stimulus are exciting television programmes, or watching distressing or emotional events on current affairs or television news programmes. These should also be avoided one to two hours before bedtime.

Bedroom

Make sure that your bedroom is conducive to sleep. The temperature should be pleasant, neither too hot, nor too cold. If light intrudes into the room blackout curtains may be necessary. Earplugs are useful if noise is keeping you awake.

Make sure that your bed is comfortable. You may rest better in cotton sheets rather than synthetic fabrics. Whether you have blankets or a duvet is a personal preference but make sure that you can relax in your bed.

Bedtime routine

Going to bed at the same time each night is important and so is a regular pattern of activity near to bedtime such as a warm bath, massage, relaxation exercises, relaxing music, etc.

Eating a *small* high carbohydrate meal before bedtime, such as a slice of toast or biscuits, can significantly increase serotonin levels in the body, reducing anxiety and promoting sleep.

Avoid lie-ins and daytime naps. If you give in to the temptation you will not be tired at bedtime.

Vitamin B12

Vitamin B12 is important for getting a good night's sleep. In two clinical trials patients who took 1500-3000mcg of vitamin B12 daily noticed improvements in their sleep. It should be taken as part of a B complex vitamin supplement.

Alcohol

Avoid alcohol – it may encourage short-term drowsiness, but its diuretic effects will probably wake you during the night.

Smoking

Smokers are more likely to suffer from insomnia than non-smokers.

Exercise

Exercise can aid sleep. Regular physical exercise is known to improve general health and well-being and promote a better quality of rest. Avoid aggressive exercise regimes, like step or aerobics. Swimming, bicycling, walking or gardening are gentler options. Don't exercise too near bedtime.

Relaxation

Learn to relax. Although you may go to sleep while watching television or reading a book, these activities may not produce a relaxation response. The physiological effects of relaxation are the opposite of those seen when you are stressed. There are several ways to achieve this and one of the most popular is progressive relaxation. Your GP may be able to refer you to a counsellor or support group.

Bedtime

When you are unwell you may not be as physically active as usual and therefore not as tired. Don't go to bed until you feel sleepy – even if it is past your usual bedtime. If you don't fall asleep within 30 minutes, get up, leave the bedroom and do something mundane. Listen to the radio, or flick through a magazine and when you feel tired try again!

Don't raid the fridge, have a cup of tea or coffee or a cigarette. These activities will certainly make you feel even more wide awake! If you are confined to bed and can't sleep – sit up, put the light on and flick through a magazine or listen to music, etc, until you feel ready to try again.

If these measures don't help you may wish to try an alternative treatment

Valerian ~ *Valeriana officinalis*

This herb has already been mentioned in chapter 1 (see page 27) as a remedy for anxiety. In higher doses valerian root is a sedative, useful where sleep disorders result from anxiety, nervousness or exhaustion and for headache or muscular pains. Valerian makes getting to sleep easier and increases deep sleep and dreaming. It does not cause a morning hangover. Patients who take valerian usually wake feeling refreshed and feeling that they have slept well.

Researchers in Germany compared a tablet containing a combination of valerian with lemon balm and the sleeping drug, Halcion. They found that the herbal pill was as good as the drug in improving patients' ability to get to sleep. However, the drug group complained of feeling 'hung over' in the mornings and had difficulty concentrating while those taking the herbal mixture had no adverse effects.

In a small trial involving 16 patients with long-term insomnia valerian was ineffective at first, but with longer term therapy (14 days with multiple doses), improvements were noted. There was a very low incidence of unwanted effects.

Two double blind controlled trials with aqueous extract of valerian (400-900mg) versus a placebo control confirmed clinically that the herb promotes good sleep quality. It decreased the time taken to get to sleep, reduced the number of times people woke during the night and increased dream recall.

Uses
- Insomnia
- Anxiety

Recommended dosage

Tablets/capsules 200mg	1-3 tabs/caps at night
Fresh herb juice	15ml at night
Dried rhizome and root	0.3-1g at night
Liquid extract (BPC 1963) 1:1 in 60% alcohol	0.3-1ml at night
Simple tincture (BPC 1949) 1:8 in 60% alcohol	4-8ml at night
Concentrated infusion (BPC 1963) 1:5 in 25% alcohol	2-4 ml at night

Hops ~ *Humulus lupulus*

Hops are more commonly recognised as an ingredient for making beer. The female strobiles of this perennial climbing plant are used for remedial purposes.

Hops have been used for centuries as a 'bitter', promoting good digestion and treating digestive ailments. They have pronounced sedative effects and can induce sleep within 20-40 minutes.

They have a marked bitter taste but if this can be tolerated large doses can be given without any unwanted effects. For this reason hops are often included in herbal sleeping tablets.

The sleep-inducing and relaxing properties of hops were discovered relatively recently when it was noted that hop-pickers tired easily, either because of the transfer of hop resin from hand to mouth or possibly through inhaling sedative chemicals.

Hops' sedative properties come from a chemical present in small amounts in fresh leaves – concentration increases as the leaves dry.

The hormone content of hops may disrupt the menstrual cycle if used regularly. Because the hormones are mainly oestrogenic they can similarly cause decreased libido in men.

Uses
- Insomnia
- Digestive disturbance

Unwanted effects
- Direct contact with the plant can cause dermatitis.
- Excess use in men can reduce libido.
- Excess use in women can disrupt the menstrual cycle.

Interactions with other herbs
- Increase the action of other sedative herbs.
- Could interact with anti-oestrogen drugs such as Tamoxifen. However this has yet to be demonstrated.

Interactions with other drugs
- Barbiturates
- Anaesthetic agents
- Anticonvulsants
- Sedatives

Contraindications

- Depression
- Pregnancy
- Low libido in men
- Patients with oestrogen dependent cancer such as breast or uterus.

Recommended dosage
May be used as a hop pillow. Fill a small muslin bag loosely with hops that are more than a year old and pin it to an ordinary pillow or place it inside the pillowcase. The chemicals that promote sleep can then be inhaled.

As an hypnotic – it is bitter and may need to be sweetened

Dried herb by infusion	1–2g at night
Liquid extract 1:1 in 45% alcohol	2ml at night
Tincture 1:5 in 60% alcohol	2ml at night

In tablet form combined with other hypnotic herbs such as Reston

Passionflower ~ *Passiflora incarnata*

The aerial parts of this plant have been used for centuries to induce sleep and relaxation without risk of addiction.

Its effect was first verified in 1920 where it was noted that, unlike with narcotics, sleep was induced with easy, light breathing.

Lutomski confirmed this in 1960. He noticed that, upon waking, patients showed no signs of confusion, stupor or depression.

Passionflower improves tone in the sympathetic nervous system in weakened conditions, and circulation and nutrition of the nervous centres. In other words it restores the normal function of both the automatic and voluntary nervous system.

Extracts of passionflower reduce spontaneous activity in mice and prolong their sleep. The herb is also used to relieve anxiety, see page 35.

65

Uses

- Insomnia

Recommended dosage

Dried herb as an infusion	0.5–2.5g at night
Liquid extract 1:1 in 25% alcohol	0.5–1.0ml at night
Tincture 1:8 in 45% alcohol	0.5–2ml at night

Lemon Balm ~ *Melissa officinalis*

No adverse effects have ever been associated with this herb. It is easy to grow in the garden and fresh leaves can be made into an infusion with a pleasant slightly lemony taste. Unfortunately, when dried, it loses its lemon flavour. Lemon balm can be taken as a bedtime drink. It is often included in over-the-counter herbal sleeping preparations – see page 52.

Uses

- Insomnia

Recommended dosage

Fresh herb by infusion	2–4g at night
Fresh herb juice	15ml at night
Liquid extract 1:1 in 45% alcohol	2ml at night
Tincture 1:5 in 45% alcohol	2–6ml at night

Chamomile Flowers ~ *Matricaria recutita*

German and Roman chamomile have a long history of use for insomnia. German chamomile is generally considered stronger and better for adults. It is covered in more detail on page 29.

Mild sedation is produced at doses of between 30-100mg/kg.

Twelve patients were investigated for heart disease with a tube inserted into the heart through a vein. After drinking a 6oz cup of strong chamomile tea 10 out of 12 patients fell soundly asleep and slept through the procedure, showing it had strong sedative effects but no adverse effect on the heart.

It is considered safe for use in pregnancy and breastfeeding.

Uses

- Insomnia

Recommended dosage

Commercially packaged teas may give disappointing results

Dried flower heads	2-8 g at night
Liquid extract 1:1 in 45% alcohol	1-4ml at night
Tincture	5 ml at night
Essential oil	2-3 drops on a sugar lump at night

4 | Fatigue

Take care of your body with steadfast fidelity.
~ Johann Wolfgang von Goethe

Fatigue is defined as having insufficient energy to carry out a task without needing to stop, rest or sleep.

It is one of the most prevalent and distressing symptoms of cancer and its treatment. Patients often find that neither rest nor sleep significantly relieves it. Unfortunately fatigue may continue to be troublesome even after treatment has been completed and you think that you ought to feel better. It is becoming one of the most important untreated symptoms in cancer patients today.

Although the problem is very real and affects the lives of many patients, it is rarely discussed and even more rarely treated. There can be other associated symptoms such as dizziness, headache, nausea and irritability.

In addition to this, as we get older our bodies have to work a little harder to maintain their equilibrium and the body its homeostasis. Naturally any illness puts a heavy burden on bodily processes, adding to feelings of fatigue.

Tiredness can also be due to other concurrent illnesses:
- Viral illness such as glandular fever/mononucleosis (Epstein-Barr virus).
- Chronic fatigue syndrome or ME.
- Hypothyroidism or myxoedema – an inadequately working thyroid gland.
- Muscular and neuromuscular disorders, such as polymyalgia rheumatica and fibromyalgia.
- Blood disorders, such as anaemia.

- Lupus
- Diabetes mellitus.
- Neurological diseases, such as Parkinson's disease.
- Heart disease.
- Kidney disease.
- Chronic stress or anxiety (see chapter 1).
- Depression (see chapter 2).
- Menopause (see chapter 13).
- Insufficient sleep.

Following is a list of drugs that commonly cause fatigue. If you are taking any of them, do *not* stop without consulting your doctor first. There may be an alternative treatment or you may be able to stop taking them altogether.

- ACE Inhibitors used for hypertension, such as Enalopril.
- Nitrates used for the treatment of angina, such as Isosorbide dinitrate.
- Benzodiazepines used either to allay anxiety or as a sleeping tablet, such as Diazepam or Temazepam (see page 18).
- Antidepressants, such as Imipramine or fluoxetine (see page 42).
- Anti-epileptic drugs, such as Carbamazepine and Primidone.
- Steroids, such as Triamcinolone and Dexamethasone.
- Beta-blockers used for anxiety attacks, thyrotoxicosis, hypertension, etc, such as atenolol, and propranolol (see page 22).
- Digoxin.
- Diuretics such as acetazolamide and frusemide.
- Statins – used for lowering cholesterol, such as simvastatin. This inhibits the enzyme HMG-CoA reductase which can cause muscle pain and weakness.
- Analgesics, such as dihydrocodeine or morphine.
- Antihistamines, such as chlorpheniramine (see page 59).

Helpful lifestyle strategies

Diet

Concentrate on eating more nutritious foods. Make sure that you are eating five helpings of fresh fruits or vegetables (excluding potatoes) daily. Some foods such as oats are known to improve energy levels. If you are not eating well discuss this with your GP or oncologist – they may recommend nutritional supplements. Occasionally sensitivity to a food such as wheat or milk can cause fatigue.

Shopping

If you can, shop over the internet and get it delivered, the small extra charge is well worth it. Your milkman may deliver bread, eggs, juice and soft drinks as well as milk. Otherwise, shop at times when it's less busy, take a list and always ask for help in a supermarket with packing and carrying the shopping to the car.

Work

Talk to your boss, she/he may be happy to re-arrange your schedule to help you. You may be able to get a parking place nearer to work or even do some work at home. It makes sense to ask to be excused heavier work when you are fatigued.

Homework

Don't feel guilty about not doing the housework when you are fatigued. Try to make just one trip down and another up stairs per day. Make a list of essential jobs and spread the tasks out over the day. Employ a cleaner if you can, you may get advice from Social Services. Take a look at your cleaning equipment, will cleaning be easier and less tiring with long handled tools or a lighter vacuum cleaner?

Childcare

If you have children, explain to them that you will not have as much energy as usual, make a game out of housework to encourage them to help at home and plan activities that you can do together while you are sitting down. Ask other parents to help with the school run when you are feeling fatigued, most will be pleased to help.

Rest

Get plenty of rest and try to stick to a regular regime. I usually suggest getting up each morning at the same time and taking some exercise, if possible, after breakfast such as stretches, yoga or a 20-minute walk. After lunch take a siesta for one to two hours, then make sure you follow a regular routine to prepare you to rest in the evening.

Exercise

It seems paradoxical to suggest more exercise when fatigue is a major problem, but a trial which looked at 72 women with newly diagnosed breast cancer over three cycles of chemotherapy showed that a regular low to moderate intensity exercise programme reduced fatigue. Patients with chronic fatigue syndrome also showed a substantial improvement in their symptoms and quality of sleep.

Dehydration

This can result in feelings of tiredness. Coffee, tea, cola drinks and alcohol do not relieve dehydration but tend to make it worse and increase feelings of fatigue. Try stopping them for a few weeks. The best way to correct dehydration is to drink six to eight glasses of water per day. If you have problems with your heart and/or kidneys consult your GP or oncologist. In any case, if this means a large increase in the amount of fluid that you drink each day I suggest building up gradually, by half a glass extra per day until you reach this level or feel that you are drinking sufficient.

Stimulants

Some herbs are sold to give more energy such as cola and guarana. These tend to be short-term stimulants and although they can give a short-term 'high', are probably best avoided in long-term illness. Recreational drugs and cigarettes should also be avoided.

Protein

Adequate protein is necessary to repair damaged tissue, produce blood, to maintain normal hormone levels and for many other biological processes. Protein is found in all meats and offal, pulses, eggs and grains.

Vitamin A

Take a vitamin A supplement. This essential vitamin continues to impress as a cancer and infection preventative. It is also necessary to promote growth and repair of mucus secreting cells and maintain cell wall strength.

Vitamin B

Take vitamin B complex – it is generally agreed that all B vitamins are useful in enhancing energy levels but two B vitamins are especially helpful:

- Vitamin B5 (also known as pantothenic acid)
- PABA (also known as para-aminobenzoic acid)

Zinc

Supplement with zinc. Low levels of this mineral interfere with blood sugar regulation, energy production and tissue repair. Zinc is also necessary for the efficient functioning of the immune system

Magnesium and Potassium

You may need extra magnesium and potassium. These two minerals are involved in just about every biological process, including production of important body proteins, regulation of glucose metabolism and release of cellular energy. They are also essential for muscle contraction and nerve conduction in the somatic muscles and those of the heart and blood vessels. Some drugs, such as diuretics (water tablets) and other treatments, deplete the body of these minerals leading to increased feelings of fatigue.

Magnesium is found in nuts, seeds and vegetables. Potassium is found in green vegetables, parsley, sunflower seeds, fish, lean meat, mushrooms, avocado and cantaloupe melon.

Coenzyme Q10

This plays an important part in the role of cellular energy production. It has been found that patients suffering from cancer have low levels of this coenzyme. Taking coenzyme Q10 has resulted in increased vitality, faster healing, improved immunity, strengthening of the heart and normalisation of blood pressure. It appears to be free of side effects. The dose is usually 30mg daily.

Spices

Any spice described as 'hot' such as ginger, cinnamon, cayenne pepper, mustard or horseradish is likely to increase blood circulation and production of chemicals in the brain that help to fight feelings of fatigue. They also improve blood supply to muscles, as well as the heart and lungs.

If fatigue persists there are plant-based medicines that have been used to enhance energy levels for hundreds of years.

Ginseng ~ *Panax ginseng*

This herb has been part of Chinese medicine for over 2000 years. It was considered so important that wars were fought to conquer lands where it grew. The root is the part used as a medicine and it is now grown commercially.

Panax comes from the Greek *panacea*, which means cure-all and ginseng from the Chinese *shin-seng* meaning man-root. There are several other herbs known as ginseng such as American ginseng (*Panax quinquefolium*), Siberian ginseng (*Eleutherococcus senticosus*), and Indian ginseng (*Withania somniferum*). These have different properties to *Panax ginseng*.

Panax ginseng has been found to increase the body's resistance to stress and noxious agents such as radiation, viral infection, tumour load, alcohol poisoning, oxygen deprivation, and temperature stress as well as movement restriction. In fact, a major virtue of this herb is its ability to make the body function 'normally'. This is called an adaptogenic action.

Panax ginseng improves physical and mental performance and has anti-fatigue effects, although some experiments failed to demonstrate this.

It may need to be taken for six weeks for you to feel the full benefits and it may work more quickly if you take it in liquid form.

Uses

- Fatigue
- To improve resistance to infection
- To improve resilience when undergoing chemotherapy
- To improve libido

Unwanted effects

These mainly occurred after prolonged use in very high doses

- Increased libido
- Breast pain
- High blood pressure
- Inability to concentrate
- Nervousness
- Skin rash
- Diarrhoea
- Insomnia
- Menstrual abnormalities
- Breast tenderness

Interactions with other herbs

- None

Interactions with drugs

- Monoamine oxidase inhibitors
- Insulin
- Warfarin
- Loop (thiazide) diuretics
- Phenelzine
- Caffeine
- General anaesthetic agents

Contraindications

- Pregnancy and breastfeeding
- High blood pressure
- Imminent general anaesthesia
- Diabetes mellitus – unless under the supervision of a physician

Recommended dosage
Standardised extract containing 4-7% ginsenosides
Tablets/capsules   100-200mg daily
Dried herb   0.5-0.8dg daily for long term use or
                   1-3g daily for short term use – up to a fortnight

Siberian Ginseng ~ *Eleutherococcus senticosus*

The root of this plant has been widely researched by the Russians. It was found to have immune stimulating effects – in healthy volunteers the level of T cell lymphocytes increased. It also showed the ability to improve endurance for Russian cosmonauts and athletes. Siberian ginseng may also assist in recovery from surgery, cancer and help patients to tolerate radiotherapy.

It is approved for use as follows by Commission E, the group of scientists who advise the German government about herbs.

As its name suggests, it is grown in Siberia and Korea but is now readily available in the UK.

Uses

- Lack of stamina
- Reduced immunity

Unwanted effects

- None

Interaction with other herbs
- None

Interaction with other drugs
- Digoxin
- Anticoagulants such as warfarin
- Insulin
- Barbiturates
- Kanamycin and monomycin – increases their effect
- Chemotherapy – women with inoperable breast cancer could tolerate more chemotherapy and/or radiotherapy.

Contraindications
- Pregnancy and breastfeeding
- Hypertension
- Diabetes mellitus

Recommended dosage
Dried herb by decoction   2-3g root daily
Tincture   1-3ml daily
Liquid extract   5-10 drops daily

Milk Vetch Root ~ *Astragalus sp.*

Astragalus is used in traditional Chinese medicine to support and enhance the immune system. It does this by stimulating antibody formation and increasing T lymphocyte proliferation.

Research in 43 patients showed that it enhanced the action of the heart and had a generalised tonic effect. It was also antioxidant and increased the breakdown of blood clots.

The herb strengthens muscle tone in the intestine, increasing movement in the digestive tract, as well as having a general protective effect on the liver.

Uses
- Lack of stamina
- Reduced immunity

Unwanted effects
- None

Interaction with other herbs
- None

Interaction with other drugs
- Cyclophospamide
- Anticoagulants such as warfarin
- Antiplatelet drugs
- Antithrombotic drugs

Contraindications
- Pregnancy and breastfeeding
- Immuno-suppressed patients
- Auto-immune disease

Recommended dosage

Capsules	2 (250-500mg), three times daily
Dried herb by decoction	2-6g root daily
Tincture	1-3ml daily
Liquid extract	4-12mls daily

Yellow Gentian ~ *Gentiana lutea*

Gentian and other herbs that are known as bitters, increase energy levels through a general tonic effect on the body. They can cause an increase in the action of the sympathetic nervous system and improvement in heart function. Muscles and nerves are stimulated and there is improved circulation to the abdominal organs, which aids their function and the absorption of nutrients.

Because they act as general stimulants some bitters have an antidepressant action, and a subtle psychological effect.

They are covered in more detail on page 104.

St John's Wort ~ *Hypericum perforatum*

Recent research has confirmed its effectiveness in treating fatigue where no organic cause can be found – see page 47.

Oats ~ *Avena sativa*

Oats have been used for centuries to improve stamina and treat general weakness and debility.

There are numerous plant steroids in oats. Avenocosides are very similar in structure and action to the ginsenosides found in Panax ginseng, responsible for its tonic and adaptogenic effect.

Oats have already been covered on page 54.

5 | Pain

I learn to relieve the suffering (Miseris succurrere disco)

~ Virgil 70BC-19BC AENEID I

Pain is probably the most frequent and most feared symptom of cancer care. Fortunately, it is not always a problem for patients who have cancer and 50 per cent do not suffer from pain at all. Not all pain suffered by people with cancer is caused by their main illness. You may experience pain from:

- Arthritis and other musculo skeletal disorders such as polymyalgia rheumatica.
- Back pain.
- An indirect consequence of the illness such as neuralgia after shingles caused by immuno-suppression.
- A direct consequence of your treatment, such as post-mastectomy, or post-thoracotomy.

For many years painkillers recognised to be most effective were derived from a plant source. Codeine, morphine and diamorphine (heroin) were originally isolated from *Papaver somniferum* – the opium or white poppy. Most painkillers are now artificially manufactured. If your pain is severe I strongly advise commencing opioid analgesia sooner rather than later. If you experience chronic or severe pain these remedies may well reduce your need for painkillers.

Relaxation
Relax, because tension always makes pain worse. A form of progressive relaxation or self-hypnosis practiced daily can cut down your need for drugs. Ask your GP or oncologist to put you in touch with someone who can teach you how to do this.

Acupuncture
Consider asking your GP to refer you for acupuncture – this is an

excellent way of relieving pain for some people. It works especially well to ease the pain of arthritis and cervical spondylosis.

Distraction
Occupy your mind. There is no doubt that distracting your attention from it can diminish pain intensity.

Ice/hot packs
Don't forget to try cold or hot packs. If pain is acute try ice first but if you have suffered the pain for a long time you may find a hot pack more comforting.

Massage
A regular massage can be very useful. An experienced masseur/masseuse can help to relax muscles made tense because of pain.

Massage oil made of hot peppers (capsaicin) can also relieve pain when massaged onto skin around the painful area.

Essential oils
Essential oil of lavender can enhance the effects of analgesics or even relieve pain itself. In the 1920s French perfume chemist René-Maurice Gattefossé burnt his hand when working in his laboratory. He plunged it into the nearest cold liquid – oil of lavender – and experienced instant pain relief. You may like to try a few drops in your bath, dripped on a pillow or cushion, or diluted with a carrier oil and rubbed directly on your skin.

Massage with some oils such as rosemary, black pepper, eucalyptus and sweet marjoram may also aid pain relief.

Diet
Some foods have natural relaxing properties. Honey and carbohydrates induce tranquillity and sleep in some people. Quercetin, found in onions, also has a relaxing effect.

Other foods, especially fruits, contain the natural analgesic, salicylate. These include apples (notably Granny Smith), oranges, sweet and hot peppers, Sharon fruit, pineapples and tea. Try to include some in your diet every day.

If you find that you still need a painkiller you could try these highly effective natural analgesics.

Devil's Claw ~ *Harpagophytum procumbens*

The root of this plant has been used in Africa for over 250 years for its anti-inflammatory properties. Devil's claw is readily available in the UK and has been shown to have an anti-inflammatory effect similar to COX II inhibitors but without the gastric upset. Unlike conventional NSAIs, which alter arachidonic acid metabolism, devil's claw alters the mechanism that regulates calcium influx in smooth muscles, thus easing pain.

It also reduces blood pressure and heart rate.

Devil's claw has a beneficial effect on stomach acid and enhances bile flow. It is licensed in Germany for dyspeptic complaints and loss of appetite as well as rheumatic ailments.

Uses
- Arthritis and rheumatism

Unwanted effects
- Headache
- Weight loss

Interactions with herbs
- None

Interactions with drugs
- Warfarin and other platelet inhibiting drugs

Contraindications
- Pregnancy and breastfeeding
- Gastritis and peptic ulcers
- Gallstones
- Diabetes mellitus

Recommended dosage
Infusion – mix 1 teaspoon of powdered herb with 300ml boiling water. Steep for 48 hrs, then strain.

Tablets – up to 2000mg daily

Cajeput ~ *Melaleuca leucadendra*

This medicinal oil is obtained from distilling fresh leaves and twigs from this tree. It smells of camphor and eucalyptus. It is ideal if you do not wish to take medicines by mouth and has a generalised rubifacient effect.

Cajeput is used on the skin only and should not be ingested.

Uses

- Arthritis
- Neurogenic pain
- Temporary relief of muscular pain

Unwanted effects

- None

Interactions with herbs

- None

Interactions with drugs

- None

Contraindications

- This oil should not be applied to the facial area. The skin is more sensitive here and dermatitis more likely to occur.
- Do not apply where there is already inflammation – in skin conditions such as dermatitis.

Recommended dosage

Dilute with a carrier oil (such as almond oil), apply to the painful area sparingly and massage in as needed.

Turmeric ~ *Curcuma longa*

This bright orange/yellow root, native to India, is a familiar spice. Its anti-cancer properties are not so well-known. Professor Will Steward at Leicester Royal Infirmary noticed that cancer rates were much lower in the Asian community and he and his team believe that long-term turmeric consumption is responsible. It may be possible to produce a supplement pill from turmeric to protect us against skin, colon and breast cancer.

Turmeric contains natural anti-inflammatory and pain-relieving chemicals especially curcumin. I have found it to be effective for musculo-skeletal pain.

It has also been shown to inhibit prostaglandin formation *in vitro* and may lower high cholesterol levels. Its anti-microbial actions are being investigated.

Uses
- Arthritis and rheumatism

Unwanted effects
- None

Interactions with herbs
- None

Interactions with drugs
- None

Contraindications
- Pregnancy and breastfeeding
- Obstructed biliary ducts
- Gallstones

Recommended dosage
Infusion of dried herb	0.5-1g, three times daily between meals
Capsules	3x 400mg daily
Tincture (1:10)	10-15 drops, three times daily

White Willow ~ *Salix alba*

For centuries a tea made with the bark of this tree was used to break fevers, soothe pains, and reduce inflammation associated with arthritis. We now know that the active ingredients include up to 12 per cent salicylic acid. It is a phyto-therapeutic precursor of acetyl salicylic acid (aspirin), which was first isolated from it in 1899. However, unlike aspirin, willow bark does not cause gastric upset, probably because of its high tannin content.

Uses

- Pain
- Neuralgia
- Arthritis and rheumatism
- Reduces fever

Unwanted effects

- None

Interactions with herbs

- None

Interactions with drugs

- Antiplatelet medication
- Warfarin
- Heparin
- Alcohol
- Barbiturates
- Non-steroidal anti-inflammatories such as Diclofenac and Ibuprofen.

Contraindications

- Pregnancy and breastfeeding
- Children
- Active peptic ulceration unless under the supervision of a doctor.
- Haemophiliacs and others with bleeding disorders.
- Asthmatics
- Diabetics

Recommended dosage

Average daily dose should correspond to 60-120mg total salicin.

Tablets/capsules	200-400mg, 2-3 hourly as needed
Infusion of dried herb	2-3g daily
Tincture (1:1)	1-3ml three times daily

St John's Wort ~ *Hypericum perforatum*

St John's wort is dealt with in detail on page 47.

It is the herb of choice for anyone suffering from shingles or any other form of neuralgia or pain emanating from nerves.

It can be used in combination with other remedies mentioned previously.

6 | Muscle cramps

The treatment with poison medicines comes from the West.
> ~ Huang Ti (The Yellow Emperor) c2500BC

There are few symptoms as unpleasant as leg cramps. These will nearly always come on at night, waking you with excruciating pain in the calf, although other muscles can be affected. Cramps usually occur during light sleep and are caused by strong muscular contractions. Very little is known about the actual cause, but over 60 per cent of people over 50 years of age have experienced them.

Rubbing the muscle vigorously can bring rapid relief. Luckily this is not a serious condition, although occasionally it can denote narrowing of the arteries of the legs and a more serious health problem called intermittent claudication. Your GP can check to make sure that you don't have this by feeling for pulses in your lower leg and foot.

Some drugs can cause leg cramps. Do not stop taking them but discuss the problem with your GP or specialist:

- Diuretics, which are often prescribed where there is fluid retention or heart failure.
- Hormone replacement therapy can cause cramps in some women (see page 161).
- Serevent, and Salbutamol (selective ß2 agonists) taken for asthma.
- Methysergide – prescribed for vascular headache (migraine).
- Beta-blockers, such as metoprolol and sotalol, taken for heart conditions or anxiety symptoms.
- Aminophylline products such as Theo-Dur, prescribed for asthma and chronic chest complaints.
- Selegiline, prescribed for Parkinson's disease.

- Donepezil – more than 5 per cent of patients experience cramps with this. It is prescribed for severe Alzheimer's disease.

- Iacidipine, prescribed for high blood pressure.

Drugs used f]or treatment

Quinine

This has been taken to relieve leg cramps for many years. It is also used as a treatment for malaria. It takes about four weeks to be effective and prevents cramps in 25 per cent of people. Quinine has a very bitter taste.

Unwanted effects

- Tinnitus, headache, flushed skin, nausea and abdominal pains.

- Occasional visual disturbance including temporary blindness.

- Blood abnormalities have occurred including intra-vascular coagulation and low platelet count (thrombocytopenia).

- Allergic reactions resulting in angio-oedema.

- Renal failure and confusion have occurred occasionally.

- Quinine should not be taken by anyone with conduction abnormalities of the heart such as atrial fibrillation or heart bloc.

- Quinine interacts with painkillers, antihistamines, anti-psychotics, cardiac glycosides, ulcer healing drugs, anti-arrhythmics – all make potential unwanted effects, especially those affecting the heart, more common.

- Some patients taking quinine have experienced low blood sugar.

- Quinine is very toxic in overdose.

Lifestyle changes which help to prevent leg cramps

Hydration

Leg cramps usually denote an electrolyte imbalance and can be caused by dehydration. Try cutting out coffee, strong tea, cola drinks, alcohol and other drinks that tend to cause dehydration and gradually increase your intake of water. Don't forget to discuss this with your GP and/or Consultant if you have heart or kidney disease.

Stretches

When you have had cramp the muscles tend to shorten, making them ache afterwards and more likely that you will have cramp again. Gently stretch each calf muscle in the morning and at bedtime by standing about twelve inches out from a wall. Place your hands flat on the wall and, keeping your heels on the ground, gently lower your face towards/against the wall. Adjust the distance from the wall until you feel a gentle stretch in the back of your leg. Continue for five minutes.

Calcium and Magnesium

You may benefit from a supplement of calcium and magnesium which is known to make muscles contract properly. You need to take a supplement with calcium and magnesium in the ratio 2:1.

Potassium

Try taking two teaspoonfuls of cider vinegar and one of honey in a glass of warm water. Cider vinegar is very high in potassium and so are most fruits and vegetables. Or substitute LoSalt (potassium chloride) for your normal kitchen salt.

Vitamin E

This is beneficial for cases of nocturnal leg cramps. Take a supplement of 1000mg of vitamin E daily.

Seaweed

Adding seaweed to your diet can help prevent leg cramps because it is high in calcium, magnesium and iodine.

If these measures don't help then here are some effective natural remedies.

Cramp Bark ~ *Viburnum opulus*

As its name suggests this is an effective treatment for cramp. The bark of this shrub is used for all types of muscular cramps including uterine cramps (period pains) and it is also an anti-spasmodic. It has a bitter taste and is easier to take as a tablet. Another herb, black haw (*Viburnum prunifolium*) can be taken as an alternative.

Uses

- Cramps

Unwanted effects

- None

Interactions with other herbs

- None

Interactions with other drugs

- None

Contraindications

- Pregnancy and breastfeeding

Recommended dosage

Tablets/capsules   6 x 200mg tablets daily
Tincture BHP (1983)   15 to 30ml daily in water

Prickly Ash ~ *Zanthoxylum sp.*

This is also called toothache bark and comes from a small, multi-branched flowering tree with impressively thick thorns. I have seen small specimens at the Eden project in Cornwall and also more magnificent subjects growing wild in Southern Africa. It works very well for muscle cramps and stimulates the peripheral arterial and capillary circulation. It also inhibits plaque formation and is included in mouthwashes in Africa. Prickly ash has a very bitter taste and some people prefer to take it as a tablet.

Uses

- Cramps
- Rheumatic pains

Unwanted effects

- None

Interactions with other herbs

- None

Interactions with other drugs

- None

Contraindications

- Pregnancy and breastfeeding

Recommended dosage

Tablets	6 x 200mg tablets daily
Tincture BHP (1983)	15 to 30ml daily in water

Black Cohosh ~ *Cimicifuga racemosa*

This has been dealt with in detail on page 174. Native Americans traditionally used it for muscle pains.

Uses

- Muscle cramps

Valerian ~ *Valeriana officinalis*

This has been covered in detail on page 27. It can be very effective in treating leg and other cramps.

Uses

- Muscle cramps of all types

7 | Indigestion

The Doctor of the future will give no medicine, but will interest his patients in the care of the human frame, in diet and in the cause and prevention of disease.
~ Thomas Edison

Most of you undergoing treatment for cancer will take drugs by mouth at some time. Unfortunately, you may suffer from abdominal discomfort throughout your treatment either as indigestion, dyspepsia, heartburn, wind or bloating. As well as being painful and unpleasant, these symptoms can be depressing and affect your progress. If you can't eat, then recovery will be delayed or compromised because you can't take in the nutrients necessary for healing to take place.

Some patients develop stomach or duodenal ulcers partly due to the medication prescribed for them and also because of the stress involved with their illness. It makes good sense to use simple remedies with low side effects to decrease this risk.

If you have a digestive upset your GP or consultant may wish to organise some tests to determine the cause.

These remedies are not meant to be a substitute for the thorough investigation of your problem.

It is imperative that you see your GP or consultant oncologist immediately if:

- You continue to feel pain, tightness or squeezing in your chest despite taking your usual effective remedy.
- You develop other symptoms such as shortness of breath, sweating, fainting, or your pain is felt in the left arm, jaw or in your back.
- Your indigestion is accompanied by changes in the frequency and/or appearance of your bowel movement.
- You are sick and there is blood in the vomit.
- You develop unexpected difficulty swallowing.

91

Many drugs can cause indigestion. These include:

- Painkillers especially non-steroidal anti-inflammatories such as Ibuprofen and Diclofenac.

- Aspirin-based painkillers.

- Chemotherapeutic agents.

- Steroids such as Prednisolone.

- Antidepressants, especially SSRIs such as Prozac (see page 42).

- Antibiotics, such as amoxycillin and erythromycin.

- Iron supplements.

- Theophylline.

- Digoxin.

Drugs can be used to treat indigestion and other digestive problems. Most of them are designed to neutralise or block acid production in the stomach. They are not always helpful because some digestive difficulties, especially in older people, are caused by insufficient acid. The acidity of the stomach is important for the first stage of digestion to occur. If there is insufficient the action of pepsin is inhibited and proper protein digestion prevented. As a result, the whole digestive process is upset, including absorption of important nutrients, essential to your recovery.

Drugs which may cause problems include:

A. Antacids containing a variety of inorganic or colloidal bismuth compounds

B. H2 antagonists such as Ranitidine and Cimetidine

C. Proton pump inhibitors, such as Omeprazole

D. Prostaglandin analogues, such as Misoprolol

E. Prokinetic agents, such as Metaclopramide

Unfortunately many of these drugs, though designed to help, can cause side effects and after coping successfully with cancer treatment the patient develops problems caused by the treatment.

A. Antacids decrease the amount of acid in the stomach. They are relatively safe for use occasionally but are known to cause the following unwanted effects if taken frequently:

- Those with a preponderance of magnesium salts can cause diarrhoea. In the presence of kidney problems they can bring about depression of the nervous system.

- Those with a preponderance of aluminium salts may cause constipation.

- There is also ever-growing evidence that aluminium may play an important role in certain aspects of brain malfunction and degenerative conditions of the brain. Some manufacturers state that insufficient is absorbed to play a significant part in neurological function. However some studies show appreciable absorption even when low doses are taken.

- Antacids containing bismuth can cause problems because it can be toxic to nerves.

- Some alkaline mixtures are strongly antacid and have a rapid effect on symptoms of indigestion, but cause acid rebound three to four hours after use. Although this may be regarded as a minor inconvenience, it may play a role in preventing ulcers and inflamed tissue from healing.

- They may interfere with the absorption of some drugs if administered with them. These include antibiotics such as Tetracycline, Ciproflovaxacin, and Ketoconazole; also Chlorpromazine, Chloroquine, Hydroxychloroquine and iron compounds.

- Some antacids cause a decrease in absorption of certain minerals such as calcium, copper, iron and phosphate.

- They may eventually cause the production of more acid.

- Antacids also interfere with the absorption of vitamins, especially B12, K, D and C.

- Long-term medication with antacids may cause the body's chemistry to become too alkaline.

- They can very occasionally cause kidney stones.

- Other uncommon side effects include headache, and co-ordination and concentration problems.

B. The histamine H2 antagonist group of drugs such as Cimetidine, and Ranitidine are designed to block production of hydrochloric acid in the stomach. This group is known to inhibit certain liver enzymes which causes an increase in the blood level of some drugs, such as Sildenafil. They are known to cause the following side effects:

- There have been rare reports of slowing of the heart and abnormalities of heart rhythm.

- They may cause skin rashes – erythema multiforme has been occasionally reported. Allergic type rashes such as urticaria are not uncommon.

- Some patients have developed confusion while taking this type of drug; others have become depressed and even experienced hallucinations.

- Changes in liver function are not unusual but generally return to normal after stopping the drug. There have been occasional reports of hepatitis, with or without jaundice. Acute pancreatitis has also been reported. This group of drugs has also caused nausea and vomiting.

- Cases of breast enlargement and discomfort have been seen in 4 per cent of users, both men and women.

- There have been some reported cases of abnormality of the blood – low white cell count and low platelet counts. This is usually reversible once treatment is stopped but more serious cases of bone marrow depression leading to serious blood abnormalities have occurred.

- Cimetidine and Ranitidine are known to affect absorption of vitamin B12 and may lead to a form of anaemia where the red blood cells are large (megaloblastic anaemia).

- Some patients have reported muscle and joint pains.

- General allergic reactions causing bronchospasm, unexplained fever, swelling and anaphylactic shock.

C. Proton pump inhibitors, such as Ompeprazole and Rabeprazole, work by inhibiting production of stomach acid. They are known to cause the following side effects:

- Nettle rash and itching in a few people. Occasionally generalised redness of the skin has occurred. These problems usually resolve on stopping the drug.

- A very few people have suffered diarrhoea. In the majority the problem disappeared after stopping treatment. Constipation, nausea, wind, dry mouth, inflammation of the lips, oral thrush, abdominal pain and vomiting have also been reported.

- Headache – in a few people this has been severe enough to make them stop treatment. In most cases it stopped when treatment ceased.

- Some patients have developed influenza-like symptoms.

- Taking this drug for a period of time has caused growth of bacteria in the stomach.

- Biochemical changes occur within the body that may have a long-term effect on health. They include decreased levels of zinc, calcium, vitamin B12, folic acid and vitamin D.

Also occasionally recorded:

- Dizziness, vertigo, light-headedness and feeling faint
- Sleepiness or inability to sleep
- Mental confusion or agitation
- Depression
- Hallucinations
- Arthritis and muscle and chest pains
- Blurred vision
- Taste disturbance
- Blocked nose
- Weight gain
- Aggression
- Swelling of feet and ankles
- Leg cramps
- Impotence
- Tingling in hands and feet

- Increased sweating
- Bronchospasm
- Increases in liver enzymes
- Fever
- Malaise
- Liver failure
- Abnormality of the kidneys resulting in acute kidney failure
- Abnormalities in the blood such as low white cells and/or platelets
- Encephalopathy in patients with pre-existing liver disease, with or without jaundice

D. Prostaglandin analogues such as Misoprolol. These have anti-secretory properties promoting healing of gastric and duodenal ulcers.

- These should not be used in women of childbearing years as they cause uterine contraction and may result in miscarriage.
- Diarrhoea may occur which can be severe and prolonged.
- Abdominal pain and dyspepsia may occur.
- Other gastro-intestinal effects such as flatulence, nausea and vomiting.
- Skin rashes.
- Dizziness has occurred occasionally.
- Vaginal bleeding, heavy bleeding and inter-menstrual bleeding have been reported in pre- and post-menopausal women.

E. Prokinetic agents such as Metaclopramide work by restoring normal co-ordination and tone to the upper digestive tract. They are widely used and the incidence of adverse effects is low. However, the following unwanted effects have been reported:

- Involuntary movement of muscles which can be alarming but usually respond to treatment.
- Drowsiness, restlessness and confusion.
- Skin rashes can occur immediately and last for up to a year after stopping medication.

- Depression has been reported very occasionally.

- Diarrhoea is also rare.

- Disorders of the red cells of the blood have been seen.

- Some patients develop high levels of the hormone prolactin –this can lead to lactation.

- Rarely a reaction called the neuroleptic malignant syndrome has been seen. This has nothing to do with cancer but is a potentially fatal reaction comprising high body temperature, altered consciousness, muscle rigidity, and other chemical changes within the body.

Helpful lifestyle changes

Smoking
If you smoke, then you should give up now – this will almost certainly improve any digestive problems. Smoking increases stomach acid production and weakens the muscle (sphincter) between the stomach and oesophagus.

Clothing
Make sure your clothes fit loosely and comfortably. Anything that constricts your abdomen – tight belts, corsets, pantie girdles or even tight jeans – can push acid upwards into the oesophagus, resulting in pain.

Meal times
Give yourself adequate time to eat. Sit down and enjoy your food and take your time chewing it. Your posture is important. If you slouch in your chair stomach contents can be squeezed upwards, making indigestion more likely.

Position
Eating just before going to bed or while in bed is not a good idea but sometimes when you are unwell it is unavoidable. If you can, sit out in a chair while you eat or sit well up in bed with your back supported. Don't lie down for at least an hour after eating.

If your symptoms are troublesome when you lay down prop the bed head up with a house brick or you may be able to borrow blocks from your local home loans department via your district or Macmillan nurse.

Don't be tempted to use an extra pillow – this will make you bend in the middle and increase pressure on your lower oesophageal sphincter.

Meal sizes

Eat smaller portions – perhaps having several small meals a day will suit you better. Although it is okay to have a light snack before bedtime, don't eat a heavy meal within four hours of retiring for the night.

Problem foods

Avoid foods that you know don't suit you. These may include spicy foods, raw vegetables, bread, pasta, potatoes and other 'stodgy' items.

Flour, sugar and salt

Decrease consumption of white flour, refined cereals, sugar and salt. These can aggravate indigestion.

Weight

If you are overweight, try to slim down as this can help reduce symptoms of indigestion and heartburn. Ask your GP or practice nurse for advice.

Saturated fats

Many people get indigestion after a meal high in saturated fats. It makes sense to examine your intake and make sure that whatever fats you do eat are beneficial to health. Cut out saturated fats (hard fats found in pastry, sausages and fatty meats) and trans fatty acids (found in margarine, biscuits, and chocolate).

Caffeine

Reduce consumption of caffeine – found in coffee, cola drinks, strong tea, chocolate and stimulant herbs such as guarana, *Cola nitida* and *Ephedra sinica*.

Alcohol

Take care with your alcohol consumption – some alcoholic drinks such as spirits and beer may precipitate heartburn or indigestion. Alcohol is less likely to cause a problem if taken with food.

Fibre

Make sure you are eating enough fibre – preventing constipation will help food to pass through the intestines, reducing the effects of reflux and heartburn. Research has shown that a high fibre diet can reduce recurrence of ulcers, gastritis and indigestion.

Cabbage

Cabbage juice has a healing effect on the mucous membrane of the stomach and intestine. You need to drink a litre per day – adding carrot juice improves the flavour.

Herbs

Some herbs can irritate a sensitive gut and it is better to avoid them. They include aloe vera, mustard seed, cayenne and horseradish. Research shows that others help to settle the stomach including tarragon, lovage, celery, chives, parsley, coriander, vanilla and savory.

Fluids

Try to drink eight glasses of water per day but not at the same time as your meals or your stomach will feel distended and you may have to eat less.

A glass of cool papaya, mango or pear juice has been shown to soothe acid burning in the oesophagus.

Acidophilus

Eat beneficial bacteria. These are similar to the bacteria that normally inhabit the healthy gut. They are usually of the genus acidophilus, lactobacillus or bifidobacterium and are considered to be beneficial because:

- They reduce the chances of harmful bacteria proliferating and causing diarrhoea. They also improve digestion.
- They make B vitamins (especially B6, niacin, folic acid) easier to absorb. Eating a cupful of live (non-pasteurised) yoghurt per day is the easiest way of taking them for most people. If you are unable to eat dairy products then acidophilus capsules are a suitable alternative.

Proteolytic enzymes

Some people have benefited from a supplement of proteolytic enzymes. Plant based proteolytic enzymes are found in small amounts in pineapples (bromelain) and papayas (papain) and also in ginger. Your GP or practice nurse should be able to advise you on whether a supplement would be appropriate.

Many natural remedies have a long history of treating these complaints safely. There is now a large body of research which confirms their effectiveness. You will find some in your kitchen or medicine cupboard.

Ginger ~ *Zingiber officinalis*

Ginger is probably better known as an ingredient in cooking than a medicinal herb. However, it is one of the most commonly prescribed medicines in the world and its effects are truly amazing and very beneficial.

In the digestive system, ginger first has an effect on the salivary glands, increasing saliva production and the amount of the digestive enzyme amylase it contains. This improves digestion at the very outset of the process. Once food is swallowed ginger calms the stomach, reduces excess acid, and stimulates normal gut movement, increasing intestinal muscle tone. As a result absorption of oral drugs is increased.

In 1973 Thompson *et al* demonstrated that ginger root contains an enzyme that aids digestion and so helps to prevent symptoms of indigestion.

Uses
- Indigestion
- Bloating
- Flatulence
- Nausea (see chapter 8)
- Vertigo

Unwanted effects
- Heartburn can occur when large doses of ginger are taken.
- Occasionally dermatitis can occur on skin in contact with ginger root.

Interactions with other herbs
- None

Interactions with other drugs

- May increase the action of drugs that decrease platelet stickiness, such as Ticlopidine and Persantin.
- May increase the action of warfarin and theoretically lead to bleeding.

Contraindications

- Gallstones
- Pregnancy and breastfeeding unless under medical supervision

Recommended dosage

0.5-1g of fresh ginger (finely sliced, bruised or grated) per cup of boiling water. Allow to infuse for 10 minutes, strain, and cool to blood heat before drinking. Take three times a day

Tablets/capsules – 2 (200mg) tablets every 2-3 hours (max 4g daily)
Weak tincture BP (1:5 in 90% ethanol) – 1.5-3ml thrice daily
Strong tincture BP (1:2 in 90% ethanol) – 0.25-0.5ml thrice daily

Preserved/crystallised ginger can also be used but is not advised for regular use because of the high sugar content

Liquorice ~ *Glycyrrhiza glabra*

Liquorice root is well recognised but its medicinal actions are probably not as well known as its usefulness in making sweets. Until relatively recently liquorice was commercially cultivated around the West Yorkshire region.

It is a very beneficial herb and its pleasant taste makes it useful to take when indigestion is troublesome. Liquorice is available in several medicinal forms, such as a tincture but natural liquorice root can be readily purchased from health food shops. Sweets are useful in an emergency situation but are not recommended for regular use because of their high sugar content.

In the late 1940s a Dutch doctor noticed that patients with gastric ulcers were cured by taking liquorice extract, dispensed by a local pharmacist. He conducted clinical trials on liquorice and found it to be effective.

Liquorice is thought to increase natural production of mucin, a substance that protects the lining of the stomach and duodenum against damage. It is also thought to increase the lifespan of gastric epithelial cells. It does not affect gastric motility or acid secretion.

- Liquorice has protective effects against gastric ulcers induced by aspirin.

- In many clinical trials liquorice was shown to accelerate healing of gastric ulcers.

- In a randomised single blind controlled trial involving 100 patients with proven peptic ulcer disease, liquorice, in the form of Caved-S, performed almost as well as cimetidine in healing stomach ulcers (88 per cent v 94 per cent).

- Liquorice has also been used in a deglycyrrhizinated form to treat gastric and duodenal ulcers.

- Liquorice appears to inhibit the growth of *H pylori*. This bacterium has been implicated in the formation of ulcers in the stomach and duodenum.

- Studies indicate some benefit in treating duodenal ulcer, with endoscopic confirmation of healing as well as symptomatic improvement.

- Liquorice has been used successfully to treat mouth ulcers.

Liquorice has a healing effect on the adrenal glands. This is very useful when patients are under great physical and mental stress. It has been shown to prevent the immunosuppressant actions of cortisone in animal studies. Although more research is needed to confirm this effect in humans, it has long been an indication for the use of liquorice in herbal medicine

Liquorice should only be used under medical supervision in patients with heart disease, hypertension, liver disease or diabetes.

Uses

- Indigestion
- Gastric and duodenal ulcers
- Aphthous (mouth) ulcers

- To prevent gastric upset in patients taking non-steroidal anti-inflammatory drugs and aspirin.
- To prevent side effects of steroid drugs and improve their action.
- As an anti-inflammatory.
- To improve the action of interferon.

Unwanted effects

- Excessive use of liquorice may cause the body to lose potassium.
- It can cause changes in body chemistry.
- Mild fluid retention may occur.

Interactions with other herbs

- *Digitalis purpurea* (Foxglove)
- *Rhamnus purshiana* (cascara sagrada)

Interactions with other drugs

Liquorice can have undesirable effects with the following:

- Corticosteroids
- Thiazide diuretics such as bendrofluazide, chlorthalidone, and hydrochlorothiazide.
- Loop diuretics such as Frusemide.
- Anti-arrhythmics, such as procainamide and quinidine.
- Digoxin
- Contraceptive pill.

Liquorice has desirable effects with:

- Aspirin
- Non-steroidal anti-inflammatory drugs such as Ibuprofen, naproxen and voltarol.
- Isoniazid
- Interferon

Contraindications

Liquorice is contraindicated in the following conditions unless under the supervision of a doctor or other qualified medical person:

- Low blood potassium
- Hypotonia
- Hormone dependant cancers such as breast and ovarian cancer.
- Diabetes mellitus
- Glaucoma
- High blood pressure
- Kidney disease
- Heart disease and stroke
- Congestive cardiac failure
- Pregnancy and breastfeeding
- Liver disease including chronic hepatitis, cirrhosis of the liver and cholestatic jaundice.
- Alcoholism
- Obesity

Recommended dosage

For indigestion, etc:

Powdered root	1-4g or by decoction thrice daily
Liquid extract BP (1973)	2-5mls thrice daily
Tincture	2-5ml three times daily

For peptic ulcers:

Deglycyrrhizinised liquorice extract BP – 0.4-1.6g thrice daily

Higher doses of treatment should be of limited duration – not more than 4-6 weeks.

Yellow Gentian ~ *Gentiana lutea*

Yellow gentian is one of a group of herbs known as bitters. Bitters are not a genus of plants but rather plant medicines from different families that all contain the bitter principle in differing amounts. They have been used extensively to treat anorexia and indigestion for hundreds of years. In Germany, gentian has been subject to intensive study for decades.

Gentian is one of the most potent of this type of herb and it is a remarkable aid to digestion. It also eliminates wind, heartburn and flatulence. Gentian can stimulate the appetite, increase saliva and digestive secretions as well as having a generally beneficial effect on the process of digestion and absorption. Because of this it should be taken about an hour before meals. Its activity begins after about five minutes when the bitter principle acts by stimulating the vallate papillae on the tongue which, in turn, stimulate secretion of digestive enzymes.

A peak is reached at 30 minutes and is maintained for two to three hours.

Gentian is also a choleretic, that is, it has an effect on bile flow, stimulating the emptying of the gall bladder, making the bile more liquid, aiding fat and protein digestion and absorption, as well as alleviating chronic constipation by encouraging gut motility.

From research and clinical experience it can be seen that gentian is a general tonic for the digestive system. Many herbalists believe that it is a tonic for all systems in the body apart from the genito-urinary tract. Its bitter taste can be unacceptable to some patients although it is possible to dilute it to an acceptable level.

Uses
- Indigestion
- Loss of appetite
- Fatigue

Unwanted effects
- Large doses may cause nausea

Interactions with other herbs
- None

Interactions with other drugs
- None

Contraindications
- High blood pressure
- Pregnancy and breastfeeding

- Peptic ulceration
- Inflammatory bowel conditions such as ulcerative colitis, and Crohn's disease.

Recommended dosage

Dried rhizome and root	0.6–2g or by infusion or decoction thrice daily
Tincture 1:5 in 45% alcohol	4ml thrice daily

Peppermint ~ *Mentha piperita var. vulgaris officinalis*

Peppermint is a well-known culinary herb commonly found growing in kitchen gardens. It is probably the best-known carminative, documented for this purpose since before Roman times. There are many different varieties such as spearmint, apple mint, ginger mint, pineapple mint, Moroccan mint, and Epicurean mint. They are interchangeable except *Mentha pulegium* (pennyroyal) which is toxic and should not be taken internally. Pennyroyal is used as a perfume and insect repellent.

Peppermint has been advocated for irritable bowel syndrome for many years but few know of its other uses or its mode of action. It can be used for acute and chronic indigestion, gastritis and enteritis.

Menthol is the main constituent obtained from peppermint although it also contains eucalyptol, limonene and methone among 100 other chemical components which vary in amount with the growth stage, cultivation method and geographical location. Fresh leaves are reported to contain as much vitamin C as oranges and more provitamin A than carrots!

Its essential oils improve gastric activity by stimulating the gallbladder and promoting bile secretion thereby reducing nausea, colic, and wind. Its action is essentially anti-spasmodic.

Peppermint leaf oils normalise gastrointestinal activity, removing flaccidity and reducing colic, which can be a problem in those people confined to bed or whose daily activity is limited.

Other actions include anti-ulcer and anti-inflammatory effects.

Peppermint can also inhibit and kill many micro-organisms that might cause problems especially in those already debilitated by illness.

Altogether some 30 pathogenic micro-organisms have been shown to be inhibited or killed by peppermint. Some deserve special mention:

- Influenza A
- Mumps virus
- Cold sore virus (*herpes simplex/genitalis*)
- Thrush (*candida albicans*)
- Staphylococcus aureus and pyogenes

Any variety of mint can also be safely used, but peppermint has the strongest action. Some people prefer to mix spearmint and peppermint in equal proportions because spearmint has a slightly sweeter flavour. If you are lucky enough to have several different varieties of mint in your garden then try different combinations until you find your favourite.

Uses
- Indigestion
- Flatulence
- Irritable bowel syndrome (see chapter 9)
- Nausea (see chapter 8)
- Diarrhoea
- Aromatic

Unwanted effects
- Abdominal discomfort

Interactions with other herbs
- None

Interactions with other drugs
- Calcium channel blockers (calcium antagonists)

Contraindications

- Allergy to peppermint or other members of the family *Labiatae*.
- Allergy to menthol
- Oesophagitis/chronic heartburn
- Gallbladder inflammation
- Biliary tract abnormalities
- Gallstones
- Liver damage
- Pregnancy and breastfeeding

Recommended dosage

1-2 teaspoons of dried herb per cup of water steeped for 10 minutes.
Strain and drink three times per day
Concentrated peppermint water (1973) – 2-4g three times daily
Peppermint oil – 0.05-0.2ml three times daily
Tincture – ¼ to 1 teaspoonful up to three times per day

Goldenseal ~ *Hydrastis canadensis*

Goldenseal root has been used by herbalists for many hundreds of years to treat gastritis and peptic ulceration. It is known to be astringent, antibacterial and anti-haemorrhagic and promotes the healing of mucus membranes in general, and the gut in particular, as well as preventing bleeding from peptic ulcers. Taken internally it increases digestive secretions, astringes the mucus membranes that line the gut, reduces gut inflammation and promotes healing of the gut wall in general.

One of the constituent natural chemicals, berberine, has been shown to inhibit *Helicobacter pylori* – a bacterium implicated in peptic ulcer formation.

Hydrastis is also active against a large number of pathogens that cause acute gastro-intestinal upset.

Uses

- Gastritis
- Peptic ulceration
- Some gut infections

Unwanted effects

- Reduced absorption of vitamin B with high doses.
- Constipation
- Abdominal discomfort

Interactions with other herbs

- *Digitalis purpurea* (Foxglove)

Interactions with other drugs

- Tetracyclines such as doxycycline and oxytetracycline.
- Digoxin
- Heparin

Contraindications

- High blood pressure and heart disease
- History of stroke
- Glaucoma
- Pregnancy and breastfeeding
- Patients with glucose-6-phosphate dehydrogenase deficiency
- Conditions where the gut is very sensitive such as IBS and inflammatory bowel disease.

Recommended dosage:

Capsules	1x125mg thrice daily
Dried herb	1.5-3g daily
Liquid extract BHC 1:1 in 60% alcohol	0.9-3ml daily
Tincture BHC 1:110 in 60% alcohol	6 to 12 ml daily

Marshmallow Root ~ *Althaea officinalis radix*

This plant inspired the soft white confectionery with which most of us are familiar. In the Middle Ages when crops failed people boiled the roots of marshmallow and fried them with onions. It contains a natural starchy substance (mucilage) that made it both nutritious and filling. Nowadays it is a frequently used herb that is both effective and safe.

This root soothes the membranes of the digestive tract. Aerial parts of the plant may also be used but they are less potent.

Marshmallow's high mucilage content makes it a soothing, healing addition to any regime for indigestion. It reduces local irritation and has been used for centuries to treat inflamed and irritated mucus membranes. It is especially useful in treating heartburn where there is reflux oesophagitis. It also stimulates the beneficial action of white blood cells.

Uses
- Heartburn and indigestion
- Reflux oesophagitis

Unwanted effects
- None

Interactions with other herbs
- Absorption of other herbs may be delayed

Interactions with other drugs
- Absorption of other drugs may be delayed

Contraindications
- Pregnancy and breastfeeding

Recommended dosage
$1/2$ to 1 teaspoonful of chopped root per cup of water. Boil gently for 10–15 minutes, cool and strain. Drink 3 cups per day.

Slippery Elm ~ *Ulmus fulva*

Many people will be familiar with this herb as a convalescent food. The tree is native to North America where Native Americans found many medicinal uses for it. The inner bark of the tree has the greatest therapeutic benefit. Slippery elm is demulcent, it increases the bulk of the stool and nourishes and heals the mucus membrane of the gut.

I find slippery elm particularly useful for patients who have heartburn/reflux oesophagitis. They should take it after food to minimise symptoms and heal the oesophageal mucosa. It is also a valuable supplement for patients taking non-steroidal anti-inflammatory drugs such as Diclofenac, where it reduces the incidence of indigestion and possibly the risk of gastro-intestinal bleeding.

Uses
- Heartburn and indigestion
- Reflux oesophagitis
- For patients taking Non Steroidal Anti Inflammatory agents like Brufen

Unwanted effects
- None

Interactions with other herbs
- None

Interactions with other drugs
- None

Contraindications
- None

Recommended dosage
Slippery elm powder can be blended with water to make a gruel. Mix 2-4 heaped tablespoons with water and yoghurt, porridge oats, stewed fruit, maple or golden syrup.

Infusion (1-2g in 200ml water)	3-4 cups per day
Tablets/capsules (400-500mg)	2-3, three or four times daily
Tincture	5ml three times daily.

8 | Nausea

The Lord has created medicines out of the earth; and he that is wise will not abhor
them.   ~ Ecclesiastes

Nausea and its accompanying symptoms of feeling sweaty, faint, dizzy, under the weather and generally out of sorts is one of the most unpleasant symptoms of numerous health problems and also the unwanted effect of a whole range of medication. The experience of vomiting that often accompanies it can be extremely debilitating. Unfortunately, nausea brought about by chemotherapy often tops the list for frequency and severity.

Nausea and vomiting can be caused by:

- Chemotherapy

- Unwanted effects of medication(s) – see later.

- Infections of the digestive tract, ie food poisoning, when it is the body's way of ridding itself of potentially harmful foods or toxins from foods.

- Inner ear disorders/motion sickness.

- Excess alcohol or fatty foods.

- Morning sickness in pregnancy.

- Emotional stress and shock.

- Raised intra-cranial pressure (pressure inside the brain).

- Bowel obstruction and other gastro-intestinal disorders, such as gall-stones.

In most cases such as digestive upset, after one bout of vomiting you begin to feel better, but sometimes the nausea persists with unpleasant and painful retching even after the stomach has been emptied. When this is prolonged it results in abdominal pain and discomfort. Very occasionally the area of the stomach that joins onto the oesophagus (gullet) can tear because the repeated trauma caused by powerful muscular contractions gives rise to bleeding – Mallory Weiss syndrome.

Your family doctor or oncologist should always be told of persistent nausea and vomiting. Further investigations may be needed as many causes such as chronic stomach ulcers or gallstones require specific and not symptomatic treatment. If you are unable to keep anything, even fluids, down for 24 hours or your vomit contains blood you should contact your GP at once.

Some drugs can make you feel sick. If you are taking any of the following drugs and experiencing nausea, contact the doctor who prescribed them for you. It may be possible to change them for another medication. Do *not* stop taking them without medical advice:

- Analgesics such as morphine
- Antibiotics such as erythromycin
- Non-steroidal anti-inflammatory agents such as Diclofenac
- Antidepressants such as Fluoxetine (see page 43)

Drugs that are prescribed to prevent nausea:

A. *Phenothiazines* – this group includes prochlorperazine, perphenazine, trifluoperazine and chlorpromazine. They act on the brain to relieve feelings of nausea.

B. *Metaclopramide* improves gut motility, encouraging stomach emptying, and therefore relieves nausea.

C. *Domperidone*

D. *Betahistine* is used mostly for nausea associated with middle ear disease. It should not be prescribed to patients with asthma or peptic ulcer.

E. *Specific 5HT3 serotonin antagonists* such as Granisetron, Ondansetron, and Tropisetron. These are used predominantly for patients on chemotherapy and should be avoided during pregnancy. Special monitoring is required if there are liver or kidney complaints.

F. *Antihistamines* such as Cinnarizine and Cyclizine can be a useful therapy.

G. *Nabilone* is a synthetic cannabinoid that is used where patients have failed to respond to other treatments. Its action is not yet fully understood.

Some of these drugs have unwanted effects, which may mean that they are not particularly helpful in dealing with nausea. Sometimes prescribed drugs don't totally alleviate feelings of nausea and most herbal remedies can be added to drug regimes.

A. *Phenothiazines* are known to cause the following:

- Sedation
- Dry mouth
- Dry or congested nose
- Blurred vision
- Constipation
- Difficulty passing urine
- Dizziness
- Low blood pressure
- Involuntary muscle movements
- Symptomatic Parkinsonism

B. *Metaclopramide*
This has already been discussed on page 96.

C. *Domperidone* is known to cause the following:

- Skin rashes and other allergic reactions.
- Acute anaphylactic reactions are rare but have occurred.
- Involuntary muscular movements.
- Reduced libido.
- Enlargement of breast tissue in either sex and/or milk production in women – this is caused by a rise in the level of the hormone prolactin.

D. *Betahistine* rarely causes unwanted effects but the following have been reported:

- Gastrointestinal upsets, including abdominal pain.
- Skin rashes – sometimes they have occurred after the drug has been stopped. Itching has also been seen.
- Headache.

E. *Specific 5HT3 serotonin antagonists* are known to cause the following:

- Constipation, because they slow down gut transit time.
- Headache is the most frequently noted unwanted effect.
- Flushing.
- Hiccups.
- Fatigue.
- Gastro-intestinal complaints, such as abdominal pain and diarrhoea.
- Changes in liver function tests.
- Some drugs in this group may exacerbate high blood pressure.
- Hypersensitivity reactions, including skin rashes are rare.
- Visual disturbance.
- Dizziness.
- Involuntary movement disorders.
- Seizures.
- Chest pain, irregular heartbeat, low blood pressure and slow pulse have been seen occasionally.
- In very rare cases collapse, fainting and cardiac arrest have been reported but the relationship with the drug has not been thoroughly established.
- Animal studies showed an increase in hepatocellular carcinoma. It is not known how this relates to humans.

F. *Antihistamines* have already been discussed on page 59.

G. *Nabilone* is known to cause the following:

- Depression of respiration especially in older people.
- Low blood pressure.
- Low body temperature.

Try these non-drug alternatives before you consider adding another drug or herb to your regime.

Diet

Take small meals if possible, more frequently. Try to make them appetising and visually appealing using colour, spices, herbs and variety of textures.

Favour savoury foods over sweet ones – although sucking bitter chocolate has been known to help nausea. Avoid fatty and stodgy food. Eat plenty of fresh fruit instead – liquidised or juiced if you prefer.

Eating dry crackers or thin crisp toast without butter can sometimes stop nausea if taken early enough. This is useful first thing in the morning or if you are away from home.

If you lose a lot of weight there are several high calorie sachet preparations, for use where food intake is limited. Ask your Macmillan nurse for advice.

Dairy products

Avoid dairy products. Nausea and vomiting can temporarily diminish your ability to digest the sugar (lactose) in milk and milk products.

Fluids

Try to take small sips of a bland or clear liquid regularly, or let an ice cube dissolve in your mouth if nausea is very persistent. Other options include apple juice ice cubes, chilled herb teas, fruit juices, ginger ale, or clear broth. Avoid diet drinks containing chemical sweeteners – sugar (sucrose) assists the body in the process of absorbing water from the gut. Although you must try to maintain an adequate fluid intake, don't drink a lot with your meal as it will fill you up too quickly and exacerbate your nausea.

Relaxing

Try not to lie down for an hour or two after eating. If you need to rest, relax in a chair or recliner. If you are in bed raise yourself on pillows.

Clothes

Dress in loose clothing made of natural fabrics like cotton or wool that allows perspiration to evaporate and keeps you cool and comfortable. Make sure clothes are not too tight and do not restrict the body.

Fresh air

A fan blowing on you, an open window or even air conditioning can reduce feelings of nausea.

Vitamin B6
Vitamin B6 is known to help – try taking a supplement of 50mg daily or foods high in this such as brewers' yeast, eggs, liver, walnuts, cantaloupe melon, wheat germ and soya beans. This vitamin works best in conjunction with vitamins B1, B2, C, pantothenic acid and magnesium.

Absorption
Some herbs are absorbed through the skin so if you don't feel up to drinking soak a clean hand towel in the herbal infusion and apply the cloth to your stomach. Another option is to add a strong infusion to your bath water and relax in it.

Essential oils
Essential oils like cardamon, sandalwood, fennel, ginger and Roman chamomile can be diluted and used as massage oil – the active principles are absorbed through the skin and may help to prevent nausea.

Some herbs have been shown to have anti-nausea effects and can be safely taken with anti-nausea drugs.

Ginger ~ *Zingiber officinalis*

The clinical studies of Mowrey and Clayson first generated a wider interest in ginger as an anti-emetic. Much research has also been carried out into its benefits in cases of motion sickness as this is the easiest form of nausea to bring under experimental control.

Mowrey and Clayson compared the effects of ginger, the anti-nausea drug, diphenhydrinate, and a placebo, on the symptoms of travel sickness in 36 healthy volunteers. Ginger was found to be superior. It works for over 90 per cent of people.

In particular, taking ginger beforehand has been shown to prevent vomiting induced by the chemotherapy drug, Cyclophosphamide.

It has also been used to reduce vomiting before day-case surgery, where it was found to be more effective than Metaclopramide (Maxolon).

Anti-nausea drugs are very effective in most cases and lead to greatly reduced nausea and vomiting. However where they are not fully effective, ginger can be safely added to the drug regime.

Powdered ginger or fresh root ginger makes a pleasant tea. Add a twist of lemon peel, sugar or honey to taste. When you feel very nauseous ginger ale, ice cold from the fridge, is most acceptable and easy to sip. Make sure it is real ginger ale and avoid artificial flavourings and sweeteners. If you prefer something dry, try nibbling a crisp ginger biscuit.

Ginger has already been discussed for use in indigestion on page 100.

Uses

- Nausea

Recommended dosage

For sickness (as an anti-emetic) – 0.5-2g single dose of powdered rhizome in tablet or capsule form 40-60 minutes before travelling. 0.2-0.4g as further doses 2 hourly.

For chemotherapy induced nausea and vomiting – 1.5 g of ginger per day in any form.

Post-operative nausea and vomiting – 0.5-2g ginger daily in divided doses.

Preserved/crystallised ginger can also be used but is not advised for regular use because of its high sugar content.

Cinnamon ~ *Cinnamomum zeylanicum/verum*

Cinnamon was used medicinally long before it became popular as a spice and flavouring. It contains phytochemicals called catechins, which have been found to relieve nausea. The essential oil obtained from cinnamon bark is antibacterial, inhibits fungal growth and is known to promote gut motility. Cinnamon also increases gastric secretions slightly, thus aiding digestion.

Uses

- Nausea
- Dyspepsia

Unwanted effects

- None

Interactions with other herbs

- None

Interactions with other drugs

- None

Contraindications

- Pregnancy and breastfeeding

Recommended dosage

0.5-1g of cinnamon bark per cup of boiling water. Allow to steep for 10 minutes and strain.

Tincture   2-4ml diluted in water three times daily
Liquid extract   1-1.5ml three times daily

Black Horehound ~ *Ballota nigra*

This herb takes its name from Horus, the Egyptian god associated with healing. It is native to most of western, central and northern Europe, and was introduced to the USA intentionally for use as a medicinal plant. Aerial parts are harvested while in flower.

It should not be confused with white horehound (*Marrubium vulgare*), which is often prescribed for coughs and other chest conditions.

Although black horehound's action has never been satisfactorily explained, it remains an effective anti-emetic.

In some European countries it is prescribed to treat nervous disorders.

Uses
- Nausea

Unwanted effects
- None

Interactions with other herbs
- None

Interaction with other drugs
- None

Contraindications
- None

Recommended dosage

Dried herb as an infusion	2-5ml three times daily
Liquid extract	1-3ml three times daily
Tincture	1-2ml three times daily

Peppermint ~ *Mentha piperata var. officinalis/vulgaris*

Peppermint is a powerful antispasmodic, relaxing muscles of the gastro-intestinal tract, including those involved in anti-peristalsis or the reversal of the normal movement of the gut. It promotes the normal propulsive action of the gut therefore reducing nausea and vomiting. There is a long tradition of using peppermint to prevent nausea.

Its uses have been fully discussed on page 106.

9 | Irritable Bowel Syndrome (IBS)

Great accomplishments are possible with attention to small beginnings

~Lao Tzu

Irritable bowel syndrome is defined as a functional gastrointestinal disorder. It is specifically characterised by abdominal pain associated with opening your bowels or by a change in bowel habit. There is no specific medical test to identify it.

Diagnosis is made by excluding other, often more serious, conditions that present with similar symptoms. These include bowel cancer and inflammatory conditions of the bowel such as Crohn's disease and ulcerative colitis. Gynaecological conditions such as endometriosis or ovarian cancer can also have similar symptoms.

The clinical features of IBS are now well established. They are:

- Abdominal pain or discomfort, made better by opening the bowels or associated with a change in frequency of opening the bowels.
- Sometimes this happens at the same time as a change in stool consistency (either constipation or diarrhoea).

Two or more of the following may occur at the same time:

- Altered frequency of opening the bowels.
- Changes in the form of the stool.
- Feelings of urgency to open the bowels, straining, or a feeling of incomplete emptying of the bowels.
- Abdominal distension or bloating.

Other symptoms are often associated with IBS. These include:

- Fatigue.
- Upper abdominal pains.
- Flushing or a feeling of faintness.

- Back pain.
- Nausea.

It follows that two people suffering from IBS may not have identical symptoms.

Over one third of the UK population suffer from some symptoms of IBS at any one time and 15 to 20 per cent have symptoms severe enough to take medical advice. In a study of family doctors' practices around Bristol, it was found that of the 3000 patients attending these surgeries 255 had a gastrointestinal problem. Of those 255, 30 per cent fulfilled the criteria for IBS. The majority of them were women and a large proportion had other health problems too.

IBS accounts for half of all reported gastrointestinal complaints and half of all referrals to gastroenterologists.

It is now thought to be part physical and part psychological in origin but there are few studies into its causes.

An attack of gastroenteritis may be a risk factor. Three hundred patients with confirmed bacterial gastroenteritis were assessed in a study lasting for one year. Statistically, they were found to be at greater risk of IBS than a control group.

Psychological factors were considered in a study of 619 patients diagnosed by their family doctors with non-specific abdominal pain. Forty per cent were thought to have IBS and also had higher levels of anxiety and depression.

Drug treatment of IBS is, in my opinion, not very successful. Several drugs marketed for its treatment have now been withdrawn from sale because of serious side effects. Alosteron reduced blood supply to the bowel leading to intestinal damage. This resulted in the death of several patients. Cisapride was withdrawn because several patients died of heart complications while taking it.

Drugs prescribed for IBS include:

A. Colofac (Mebeverine)

B. Alverine (Spasmonal)

C. Dicyclomine (Merbentyl)

D. Hyoscine (Buscopan)

E. Metaclopramide (Maxolon)

Unwanted effects

A. Colofac is not known to have any significant unwanted effects.

B. Alverine is known to cause the following:

- Nausea
- Headache
- Dizziness
- Itchy rash
- Allergic reactions, including anaphylactic shock.

C. Dicyclomine is known to cause the following but all occur seldom:

- Dry mouth and thirst
- Dizziness
- Fatigue and sedation
- Skin rash
- Constipation
- Lack of appetite
- Nausea and vomiting
- Headache
- Pain on passing urine

D. Hyoscine is known to cause the following:

- Dry mouth
- Blurred vision
- Constipation
- Anorexia
- Nausea and vomiting
- Pain passing urine
- Fatigue

E. Metaclopramide has already been discussed on page 96.

These non-drug strategies may help:

Fibre
Although an increase in fibre can be useful for many people with IBS, a number of sufferers are sensitive to wheat in any form including wheat bran.

Rye, oatmeal, barley and brown rice are also high in low allergy fibre and may be eaten regularly. Psyllium husk (see page 131) may be preferred.

Food allergies
It is now believed that food allergies play a large part in this problem. Your GP, nutritionist or practice nurse can advise you.

Caffeine
Avoid drinking caffeine-containing beverages. For some people caffeine is a powerful drug, which can stimulate, even over-stimulate, the bowel causing colic and diarrhoea. Caffeine is found in coffee, chocolate, strong tea and some herbs such as *Ephedra sinica*, *Paullina cupana (guarana)*, and *Cola nitida*.

Acidophilus
Eating beneficial bacteria such as acidophilus in the form of natural yoghurt or capsules can be helpful if you are unable to eat dairy produce. This is especial useful if IBS followed an acute bowel infection or taking antibiotics.

Lactose
If you experience diarrhoea you may be sensitive to the lactose in milk and other dairy products. Try excluding all forms of dairy produce from your diet. If this is helpful you may be able to reintroduce lactose reduced milk, cream, butter and cheese without recurrence of symptoms. Rice milk and soya milk may be suitable alternatives.

Psychologists
Hypnosis may be beneficial. Your GP will be able to advise you.

Other psychological therapies have been used with varying degrees of success. These are most likely to help if you feel very anxious or distressed about your symptoms. Although stress does not cause IBS, it can make it worse and many patients benefit from practising relaxation therapy and yoga.

Your family doctor may suggest referral to a psychologist or counsellor. Multi-component behavioural therapy, including education, relaxation techniques and problem-solving strategies have been found to be superior to drug therapy alone in treating IBS.

Many herbs can be helpful, including the following:

Peppermint ~ *Mentha piperita*

Peppermint is probably the best-known carminative. It has been advocated for irritable bowel syndrome for many years and has other beneficial effects on the gut. Some researchers have found that enteric-coated tablets of peppermint work better than capsules because they pass through the stomach, unaffected by the acid environment, and only dissolve and become effective once in the alkaline environment of the small bowel. Peppermint is well- known as an antacid. See also page106.

In a recent study of 110 patients with IBS, half were treated with capsules of oil of peppermint three to four times daily, and the other patients received placebo tablets. Oil of peppermint decreased abdominal pain by 79 per cent, (v 43 per cent of controls), and abdominal distension by 83 per cent (v 29 per cent of controls). Other symptoms, such as flatulence, also improved.

Uses

• Antispasmodic

Cinnamon ~ *Cinnamonium zeylandicum*

As well as being one of the world's best known spices cinnamon is an ancient herbal medicine, used in Egypt from the 5th century BC. It is a traditional remedy for digestive upset, being antispasmodic and carminative. See page 119.

Cinnamon is also anti-viral, supporting and strengthening the gut, and can relieve diarrhoea, indigestion, nausea, wind and colic.

Cinnamon is an effective antibacterial agent, supporting its use in IBS which occurs following gut infections.

Uses

- Irritable bowel syndrome/colic
- Nausea
- Flatulence
- Diarrhoea
- Digestive upset

Chamomile ~ *Matricaria recutita*

Chamomile acts as a carminative because it is antispasmodic – easing cramp, bloating and distension, as well as toning the digestive tract. It also calms and relaxes so it is very useful if you are suffering from anxiety and stress. It is used for a large number of bowel problems and anxiety states. See pages 29 and 66 for more information.

Uses

- IBS
- Anxiety

10 | Constipation

Give me but one firm spot on which to stand and I will move the earth.
~ Archimedes (c287-212BC)

Constipation is characterised by infrequent bowel evacuations, hard, small faeces or difficult, painful defaecation. Bowel movements vary from one person to another so there is a large range of what can be considered normal. Some people open their bowels less often than others and it is perfectly normal for them.

However, if you are unwell, perhaps not taking as much exercise as usual, eating less and maybe also taking painkillers or iron tablets, onset of constipation is not unusual. Eighty-seven per cent of patients taking morphine painkillers by mouth will become constipated and 64 per cent of those taking other types will also have a problem. This compares with 20 per cent of older people who become constipated spontaneously.

Constipation is also more common as we get older, because of decreased appetite, usually as a result of lower energy needs and decline in muscle mass or if you have an illness such as depression. A change in social circumstances like living alone can reduce your motivation to prepare and eat meals. You may well have less money to spend on food, which might influence the type, quality and quantity that you buy. Sometimes physical changes occur that make shopping, cooking, chewing and swallowing more difficult.

It is important to take action early to stop it becoming a problem that will affect quality of life – perhaps causing abdominal pain, nausea, haemorrhoids, etc.

Some health problems are associated with a tendency to constipation:

- Hypothyroidism (myxoedema) – a reduction in thyroid activity.
- Depression
- Hypercalcaemia – excess levels of calcium.

Some drugs can cause constipation. Do not stop taking these but discuss them with your GP or oncologist who may be able to suggest a regime to minimise your problems:

- Painkillers, particularly morphine-based but all painkillers have a tendency to cause constipation.

- Non-steroidal anti-inflammatories, including aspirin.

- Iron tablets such as ferrous fumarate, and ferrous sulphate.

- Calcium channel blockers, especially verapamil.

- Antidepressants, such as amitriptyline (see page 42).

- Antihistamines (see pages 59).

- Over-the-counter antacids, such as aluminium hydroxide or calcium carbonate.

- Antidyskinetics, used to treat Parkinson's disease.

Non-drug ways to help

Fluids

Drink plenty of water or herbal teas such as Fennel. Try to manage two litres throughout the day. If you have a low fluid intake, perhaps because of nausea or to avoid visiting the lavatory so often, constipation is more common. Consult your nurse, family doctor or specialist before dramatically increasing your fluid intake if you have problems with your kidneys or heart. It is particularly important to increase your fluid intake if you are warmer for any reason, such as being in a warm room, or having a temperature (fever).

Dehydration

Avoid alcohol and coffee as these have an overall dehydrating effect and tend to make the stool hard and painful to pass.

Tea

Avoid drinking tea if constipation is a problem. High tannin levels can bind the stool and hold back bowel movements.

Fibre

Make sure you are taking enough fibre in your diet. Wholegrain foods such as wholemeal bread, pulses (peas, baked beans, red kidney beans, etc), fibre-rich fruit and vegetables help to prevent constipation. Studies show a lower incidence of constipation in vegetarians. In the UK frequency of consumption of fruit, vegetables and bread declines with age making constipation more likely, although there is no change in fibre requirements as you get older.

Vitamin C
Take a vitamin C supplement. This acts as a natural laxative in some people. Start with 1000mg per day and increase the dosage by 500mg per day until your bowels work. Be careful when buying supplements as many have unwanted additives such as colourings and aspartame. If you are having any hospital tests remember to tell your consultant that you are taking vitamin C as this can mask the presence of blood in the stool and alter other laboratory investigations.

Exercise
If possible take some gentle exercise. Activity stimulates bowel movement and those who are confined to bed or who rarely get up and move about are more prone to constipation.

Magnesium
Low magnesium levels can make muscles, including those of the bowel, sluggish. Try adding foods high in magnesium to your diet. Good sources are nuts, blackstrap molasses, wholegrains, soya and seafood. If these are not to your taste, take a supplement of 300-500mg of magnesium balanced by 600-1000mg of calcium.

Diet
Some foods seem to be better at gently stimulating normal bowel activity than others. Try to include at least one of the following with each meal – almonds, apples, grapes, mangoes, papayas, onions, chicory, parsley, dates, endive, figs, rhubarb, beans, turnips, walnuts, pineapples, prunes, and watercress.

Treatments
Bulking agents such as methylcellulose or bran. Bran is not suitable for everyone especially those with an intolerance to wheat. Iron, zinc and calcium are not absorbed from the gut as readily as normal in the presence of large quantities of bran because of the presence of chemicals called

phthalates. Phthalates bind these minerals preventing their absorption into the body.

Stimulant laxatives such as bisacodyl and Docusate sodium irritate the intestinal lining and prompt bowel movement.

Stool softeners, such as arachis oil and liquid paraffin allow the stool to absorb more water, making it easier to pass. They will be most useful where the patient is not able to take bulk in their normal diet.

Osmotic agents such as lactulose keep water in the intestines and thereby soften the stools.

Enemas, usually phosphate, irritate the rectum and prompt emptying.

If you need help to move your bowels and prefer herbal products, the following are known to work:

Bulk laxatives
These laxatives, whether natural or synthetic, increase the bulk of the stool and research shows that they increase the frequency of bowel movements by one to two per week. They may be better tolerated than other laxative products – patients experience less griping and other gastro-intestinal symptoms.

Psyllium Seed ~ *Plantago ovata*

This is one of the safest, gentlest laxatives there is. It has been used for this purpose for over 500 years, so its beneficial effects are well known. The dried, ripe seeds and their husks are used medicinally – they are very small and sometimes called flea seeds. These consist of over 30 per cent mucilage and add useful fibre to the diet.

When soaked in water the seeds swell in size and their volume increases. The husks form a gelatinous mass, increasing the bulk and volume of the faeces and keeping it hydrated. This increase in bulk promotes peristalsis – as they swell they press on the gut wall stimulating bowel movement. This is especially suitable for those patients who require more fibre in their diet and are sensitive to wheat bran.

Psyllium also provides some relief from painful, itching haemorrhoids. The seeds should be swallowed whole and swallowed with a large volume of water otherwise they are ineffective. You can sprinkle them onto porridge, muesli, yoghurt or cereals, or any food that you like. They should be taken with half a pint of liquid to allow them to absorb the liquid and swell to their full volume.

Theoretically, faecal impaction could occur if insufficient water is taken with psyllium. Although this has never been recorded it is probably advisable to be cautious where fluid intake is limited.

Psyllium's ability to slow intestinal absorption of sugar has been used as an aid to blood sugar control in diabetes.

Uses
- Constipation
- Diarrhoea
- Bleeding and itching haemorrhoids

Unwanted effects
- As with other bulk laxatives, some flatulence and bloating may occur in the first few days of treatment
- Allergic reaction

Interactions with other herbs
- None

Interactions with other drugs
- Lithium
- Absorption of other drugs could be impaired
- Insulin – the dose may need to be lowered

Contraindications
- Asthma – there have been several reports of allergic reaction
- Intestinal obstruction
- Faecal impaction
- Senile megacolon and other types of bowel atony
- Inflammatory conditions where the bowel is extremely sensitive, such as IBS.

Recommended dosage

3-10 tablespoons per day for chronic constipation

1-3 tablespoons per day for more acute onset of symptoms. (Increasing the dose gradually may be more helpful for some people.)

Linseed (Flaxseed) ~ *Linum usitatissimum*

This crop, with its characteristic pale blue flowers, is increasingly grown in the UK. Its use goes back for centuries and its proper name refers to the fact that the Romans recognised its versatility (*usitatissimum* = most useful).

Linseed can be taken on its own or added to cereal, porridge or muesli. As with all high fibre seeds, adequate amounts of water must be taken to keep them moving through your system. An added benefit of this treatment is that it contains significant quantities of omega 3 essential fatty acids.

Grind the seeds for best effect then keep any unconsumed seed in a refrigerator to prevent the oils from turning rancid. You can prepare two or three days' supply at a time.

Uses

- Constipation

Unwanted effects

- As with other bulk laxatives some flatulence and bloating may occur in the first few days of treatment

Interactions with other herbs

- None

Interactions with other drugs

- Absorption of other drugs may be delayed

Contraindications

- Intestinal obstruction
- Faecal impaction
- Senile megacolon and other types of bowel atony

Recommended dosage

1 teaspoon of ground seed in 1250ml water or juice up to three times daily
It can also be sprinkled on porridge, cereals or yoghurt

Bitters

These act as a general tonic for the bowel, improving tone and mobility as well as promoting bile flow. Yellow gentian is covered in detail on page 104.

Natural laxatives which contain anthroquinones:

Senna ~ *Cassia angustifolia*

This is a strong herbal stimulant laxative. The pods of the plant are generally used, but sometimes the leaf is available. This is not considered to be as strong as the pods.

Senna's effect is caused by natural compounds called sennosides, which are anthroquinones. These compounds inhibit absorption of water and electrolytes from the colon, and stimulate secretion of chloride ions. This increases the volume in the gut and the pressure of the intestinal contents, stimulating colon motility and increasing propulsive contractions.

Senna is recommended where easy defaecation is highly desirable such as in cases of anal fissure, haemorrhoids and after rectal or abdominal surgery, as well as for bowel clearance before surgery and in diagnostic investigations.

Uses

• Constipation

Unwanted effects

• Colicky abdominal pains
• Diarrhoea
• Electrolyte imbalance/low potassium levels
• Chronic use may interfere with calcium absorption

Interactions with other herbs

- *Glycyrrhiza glabra* (Liquorice root)

Interactions with other drugs

- Thiazide diuretics
- Steroids
- Digoxin
- Non-steroidal anti-inflammatories
- Calcium channel blockers
- Oestrogen

Contraindications

- Pregnancy and breastfeeding – unless recommended by a doctor or midwife.
- Conditions where the gut is very sensitive such as IBS, or inflammatory bowel disease.

Recommended dosage
As Senokot – 1-2 heaped 5ml teaspoons of granules or 2-4 tablets
As an infusion – 3-6 pods (Alexandrian) or 4-12 pods (Tinnevelly), steeped overnight in warm water
Liquid extract BPC (1973) – 0.5-2ml in water

Cascara Sagrada ~ *Rhamnus Purshianus*

Cascara sagrada is the most popular laxative in the world. It was widely used by the Native American people and introduced into Europe in the 19th century. The name Cascara sagrada means 'sacred bark'. Its action is much gentler than that of its cousin alder buckthorn. It is also said to improve bowel tone but, like all laxatives, it should not be taken regularly.

Uses

- Constipation

Unwanted effects

- Nausea, vomiting and stomach cramps
- Diarrhoea
- Fluid retention
- Electrolyte imbalance/low potassium levels
- Nephropathy

Interactions with other herbs

- *Digitalis purpurea* (Foxglove)
- *Glycyrrhiza glabra* (Liquorice root)

Interactions with other drugs

- Anti-arrhythmics
- Cardiac glycosides
- Corticosteroids
- Digoxin
- Indomethacin
- Thiazide diuretics

Contraindications

- Chronic gastrointestinal disorders
- Colitis
- Ulcers
- Haemorrhoids
- Irritable bowel syndrome
- Pregnancy and breastfeeding

Recommended dosage

Do not take cascara for longer than 14 days at a time. Prolonged and continuous use can lead to 'lazy bowel syndrome' – inability to open the bowels without chemical stimulation

Boil 1 teaspoon of well-dried bark in 3 cups of boiling water for 30 minutes. Cool, and drink 1-2 cups a day before retiring.

Tincture – ½ teaspoonful before retiring.

Aloes ~ *Aloe barbadensis*

Aloe vera seems ubiquitous nowadays. It has even found its way into detergents, although it has been used in cosmetics and shampoos for years.

Underneath the inner surface of the leaf's skin is a yellow latex or sap. This contains, among other constituents, anthraquinone glycosides which exert a powerful laxative action. The anthraquinones are split by the bacteria in the large bowel to form other molecules (aglycones). They irritate the bowel and cause intestinal secretion of water and electrolytes and improve intestinal motility. This action usually occurs about eight hours after consumption.

I recommend this herb only as a last resort in more chronic cases of constipation.

Uses

- Constipation

Unwanted effects

- Abdominal pain
- Albuminuria/haematuria, possibly due to nephropathy
- Cardiac arrhythmia
- Fluid retention with or without electrolyte imbalance

Interactions with other herbs

- *Glycyrrhiza glabra* (Liquorice root)

Interactions with other drugs

- Cardiac glycosides
- Anti-arrhythmics
- Thiazide and loop diuretics
- Corticosteroids
- Aloe may also impair absorption of other drugs because of its high content of hydrocolloidal fibre.

Contraindications

- Pregnancy and breastfeeding
- During menstruation
- Renal or cardiac disease
- Conditions where the gut is very sensitive such as IBS, or inflammatory bowel disease.

Recommended dosage

Aloe vera juice – 2-5 tablespoons twice daily.

11 | Haemorrhoids

The part can never be well unless the whole is well ~ Plato

It seems sensible to follow the chapter on constipation with one on haemorrhoids as this is the commonest cause of them.

To understand how haemorrhoids or piles develop you must consider the anatomy of the lower bowel or rectum. This is the part of the colon that leads to the anus and hence to the outside.

At the anorectal junction about 2cm above the anus there is a remarkably large complex of veins. These can be seen in the wall of the rectum by using a rectal speculum. When the rectum is full and we need to open our bowels these veins become congested and hence the message to visit the lavatory reaches the brain. Usually when the rectum is emptied they return to their normal size. But under some conditions they do not and the resulting varicosities are known as haemorrhoids, which are caused:

- When constipation occurs and there is increased dilatation of the veins.
- When excessive straining occurs and the veins are pushed downwards and displaced from their normal position.
- When pressure in the lower abdomen remains high, for example when there is an abdominal mass such as in pregnancy and during labour, or with some pelvic tumours.
- By standing or sitting for long periods which can aggravate them.

Haemorrhoids can be subdivided into internal and external. Internal haemorrhoids, as their name suggests, are inside the anus – it is not possible to see them. These are most typically noticed as blood covering the motion, blood in the toilet bowl or a blood on the toilet paper. If you see blood in your motion do not assume that you have haemorrhoids – you must see your GP who will examine you.

139

Internal haemorrhoids may be displaced or prolapsed when they descend through the anal opening, which then closes trapping them so that they gradually fill with venous blood. These are usually noticed as a painful lump at the anal margin and are then known as external haemorrhoids. They tend to itch and bleed and make maintaining personal hygiene difficult.

Some drugs tend to make haemorrhoids worse, usually those that cause constipation (see chapter 10). The usual methods of treatment are surgical.

Non-drug ways to help:

Avoid constipation
It is essential to avoid constipation if you are suffering from piles. No one knows exactly what causes haemorrhoids but 'straining at stool' makes it more likely that you will suffer from them. See chapter 10 for more information.

Fibre
Eat more fibre. Include in your diet foods like wholemeal bread, fruit and vegetables, pulses, nuts and seeds. Avoid wheat bran as this contains phytates which link with zinc, calcium and iron in the gut preventing their absorption. Psyllium seeds (see page131) have been shown to relieve constipation and to ease itching and inflamed haemorrhoids.

Fluids
Drink more to help soften stools and move food through the digestive tract. Avoid drinks containing caffeine and alcohol as these tend to cause dehydration and constipation. Try to increase the amount of water that you drink gradually until you feel that you are drinking enough.

Exercise
Exercise helps to keep your bowels regular. Any form of brisk exercise, such as a fast walk, helps to tone the abdominal muscles which in turn help to ensure regular bowel movements.

Dairy products
Eat less dairy products like milk, cheese, ice cream and white chocolate. Some people find that these foods make them constipated.

Spices
Avoid hot spices like chilli, pepper and horseradish because they may aggravate haemorrhoids. Don't forget that what burns going in also burns coming out!

Coffee
Both coffee and decaffeinated coffee can make haemorrhoids flare up because they contain oils that can't be digested and irritate the rectal mucosa. Cola drinks may also aggravate haemorrhoids.

Alcohol and cigarettes
These both can make haemorrhoids worse.

Don't take too long on the toilet
Don't be tempted to read the newspaper while sitting on the toilet. The position, with knees up and legs open, can cause slippage of haemorrhoids and, whether you are constipated or not, they will tend to prolapse.

Toilet paper
Wiping the area with scented toilet paper can severely aggravate haemorrhoids, so use a plain variety, with no perfume, no colour, no chemical additives whatsoever. Sometimes wiping with baby lotion-impregnated tissues or baby wipes minimises friction and cause less trauma.

Bidet
After wiping yourself it is quite difficult to make sure that you are clean. A bidet is very useful because you can rinse yourself after opening your bowels. It can also be used to wash before bed, reducing infection and cutting down itching.

Warm baths
Try taking a warm bath for 10–15 minutes several times a day. This relaxes the anal sphincter and allows any prolapsed piles to recede,

Keep dry
When piles are inflamed and tender it is quite difficult to dry yourself after washing. Use a cool hairdryer carefully to give yourself a blow dry. Use caution though – water and electricity do not mix, so it is safer to do this

in the bedroom. When you are dry apply a little powdered cornflour or other powder to your bottom to keep it that way.

Cream
Applying petroleum jelly or zinc oxide cream will reduce the pain and swelling of haemorrhoids, as well as making them feel more comfortable.

Cool it
If you have an acutely inflamed or prolapsed haemorrhoid, try putting an ice-cube in a plastic bag, wrapping it in a layer of tissue, then placing it on the haemorrhoid for a few minutes. It may shrink it down sufficiently for it to be carefully replaced in the rectum.

Several herbs are renowned for their effectiveness in treating haemorrhoids:

Butcher's Broom ~ *Ruscus aculeatus*

The root and rhizome of this plant are used medicinally. In animal tests they increased venous tone in capillary walls. Butcher's broom has a powerful haemostatic action, as well as being anti-inflammatory.

Butcher's broom can help to reduce itching and burning.

It is approved by Commission E for the treatment of haemorrhoids.

Uses
- Haemorrhoids
- Venous conditions

Unwanted effects
- None

Interaction with herbs
- None

142

Interaction with drugs
- Anticoagulants
- α-blockers used in benign prostate disease and hypertension
- MAOI-type antidepressants

Contraindications
- Pregnancy and breastfeeding

Recommended dose
Capsules – 100mg three times daily

Pilewort ~ *Ranunculus ficaria*

This is also known as lesser celandine, one of the first flowers of spring. It has golden yellow flowers and fleshy cylindrical roots that are said to resemble piles. Extended skin contact with the freshly harvested, bruised plant can result in skin irritation. This effect is lost when the plant is dried.

Pilewort is specifically used for non-bleeding or itching piles and can be applied as an ointment. It also soothes other itching mucus membranes.

Uses
- Haemorrhoids

Unwanted effects
- None

Interaction with herbs
- None

Interaction with drugs
- None

Contraindications
- None

Recommended dose
Applied as a cream/ointment

Chickweed ~ *Stellaria media*

This is an ancient English remedy for chronic skin conditions. Herbalists often prescribe it as a remedy for inflammatory skin disorders as it is very active in reducing itching and irritation. A cream made from it has a cooling effect and is very healing.

I often substitute it for steroid creams in eczematous or itchy conditions.

Uses
• Haemorrhoids

Unwanted effects
• None

Interaction with herbs
• None

Interaction with drugs
• None

Contraindications
• Pregnancy and breastfeeding

Recommended dose
As an ointment applied liberally to the inflamed area.

Horse Chestnut Seed ~ *Aesculus hippocastanum*

This stately tree was introduced to Britain by the Romans and, as its name suggests, was primarily used as fodder for horses and also to treat coughs in horses.

The seeds or leaf are used medicinally. The seeds act to strengthen the skin cells and improve the elasticity of blood vessel walls. They also have an anti-exudative, tightening effect on blood vessels. Horsechestnut is widely used to treat varicose veins and is licensed in Germany to treat chronic venous insufficiency. It may also be helpful in relieving nocturnal leg cramps and swelling of the legs.

Uses
- Haemorrhoids
- Varicose veins

Unwanted effects
- Nausea

Interaction with herbs
- None

Interaction with drugs
- None

Contraindications
- Poor renal or liver function

Recommended dose
Available as liquid and solid preparations for internal use and creams and gels for external use

Tablets/capsules	40-120mg daily
Tincture 1:10	0.6ml three times daily
Gel/cream	1-2% applied topically several times daily

Witch Hazel ~ *Hamamelis virginiana*

This shrub is native to North America and the leaves and bark are used medicinally to stop bacterial growth and for their unique effect on mucus membranes where it reduces swelling by coagulating proteins, increasing resistance to inflammation and at the same time it lays down a protective coating. Witch hazel can be very beneficial for haemorrhoids because it reduces infection as well as relieving painful swelling of the tissues.

The plant's effectiveness is probably a result of its astringency, also its content of volatile oils such as eugenol and carvacol.

Uses

• Haemorrhoids

Unwanted effects

• None

Contraindications

• None

Interactions with other herbs/drugs/vitamins

• None

Recommended dosage

Cream	Apply three times daily to the affected area
Suppositories	Insert one after defaecation and at night
Compress	A decoction (5-10g herb per 250ml water) may be applied locally to prolapsed haemorrhoids

12 | Skin complaints

A bundle of Myrrh is my well-beloved unto me ~ Song of Solomon 1:13

There are many different skin diseases, but here I will deal with commonly occurring problems associated with cancer and its treatment.

Aloes ~ *Aloe barbadensis*

The benefits of using aloe vera on the skin have been known for centuries. The Greeks and Egyptians revered its effects. Alexander the Great grew it in wagons so that he could carry fresh supplies on his military campaigns because of its exceptional healing properties. But once the main centres of civilisation moved to cooler northern climates it failed to grow and its benefits were largely forgotten except in tropical or sub-tropical climates. In Mexico, for example, a plant is encouraged to grow near the door of people's houses for first aid use.

The plant's sap is anti-inflammatory and stops itching. It is used for burns, scalds and other superficial skin injuries. Aloe vera has proved to be extremely effective in treating radiotherapy burns. I find the gel is most soothing if stored in the refrigerator before use.

Aloe vera has been thoroughly analysed and shown to contain over 200 substances including many vitamins.

Aloe vera has been shown to kill *candida albicans* (thrush). It has also been found to have antibacterial effects on four strains of methicillin-resistant staphylococcus aureus (MRSA).

Twenty-seven patients suffering from burns were treated on one area with aloe vera gel and Vaseline gauze on another. The area treated with aloe vera had earlier skin re-growth and the average time to complete healing was 11-12 days compared to 18 days for the Vaseline treatment. Unwanted effects, including stinging and irritation, were minor.

In a double blind, placebo-controlled trial aloe vera gel was evaluated to see if it prevented skin burns caused by radiotherapy. One hundred and ninety-four women used aloe vera gel prior to radiotherapy of the chest wall for breast cancer. Aloe vera did not prevent radiation dermatitis although its use afterwards did lead to quicker resolution of the burn induced by the therapy.

Aloe vera can also be taken internally (see page 137).

The main topical uses are

- Minor burns and scalds including burns due to radiotherapy
- Intertrigo (inflammation occurring in moist skin folds)

Unwanted effects

- None

Interactions with other herbs/drugs/vitamins

- None

Contraindications

- Known sensitivity to the plant or its derivatives or to other plants of the *Liliaceae* family.

Recommended dosage

Apply topically as needed – usually a minimum of twice daily but may be applied hourly if required.

Myrrh ~ *Commiphora mol mol*

Myrrh is familiar to us as one of the gifts brought by the Wise Men to the infant Jesus. The Egyptians used it for its antiseptic properties and also in the embalming process. Early records show that Queen Hatshepsut, Pharaoh of Egypt, sent a large army to the land of Punt, a journey of hundreds of miles, (Punt was situated on the East coast of Africa below where Mozambique is today) to bring back 33 myrrh sapling trees to plant near the temple.

Myrrh in its medicinal form is the sap of the tree dried to form a yellowy resin. It is insoluble in water and the resin is usually dissolved in alcohol. It can either be applied to the skin directly or diluted in equal quantities of hot water and allowed to cool.

It is one of the best antiseptic/antibacterials that I have ever used and successful in treating a wide range of skin infections. It is most useful for localised skin infections such as paronychia (inflammation around a fingernail), furuncles (boils), intertrigo and athlete's foot.

Its anti-viral action helps to heal cold sores and also makes it a useful gargle for sore throat, oral thrush or gum disease.

The main topical uses are:
- Cold sores (*Herpes labialis*)
- Shingles (*Herpes zoster*)
- *Herpes genitalis*
- Mouth ulcers
- Sore throats
- Gum problems and toothache
- Superficial skin infections – furuncules, paronychia, intertrigo.
- Athlete's foot and other fungal infections of the skin.

Unwanted effects
- None

Interactions with other herbs/drugs/vitamins
- None

Contraindications
- Known sensitivity to the plant or its derivatives

Recommended dosage
Myrrh may be applied as tincture, cream or essential oil.

Apply topically twice daily for skin infections such as furunculosis, and paronychia.

Apply neat tincture hourly with a cotton bud for herpes infections or dilute with equal parts boiling water and allow to cool before application. Dilute 5ml tincture in 100ml water and use as a mouthwash for gingivitis, mouth ulcers and as a gargle for sore throats.

Tea Tree ~ *Melaleuca alternifolia*

Tea tree oil is the essence produced by distillation of the leaves of the tree *Melaleuca alternifolia*. This is now a familiar product but is a relative newcomer to the UK herbal pharmacopoeia. It is extremely well used and thoroughly researched in its native Australia. Clinical trials there have shown it to be of low toxicity but very effective in treating a wide range of infectious conditions even when diluted down to one part per hundred.

The effectiveness and low allergy profile of tea tree oil depend on the ratio of two natural chemicals it contains. There should be high levels of terpene-ol and low levels of cineol.

It can be used directly as an antibacterial, diluted in bath water, and also used as a disinfectant. Clothes, sheets and towels can be washed in hot water with tea tree oil added.

Much research has been carried out into the anti-microbial and anti-fungal properties of this oil and some of the outstanding results are:

Rapid healing without scarring when tea tree oil was applied at full strength to boils two or three times daily.

Athlete's foot was either eradicated or improved in 58 of 60 subjects.

A double blind study in the *Journal of Family Practice* in 1994 found that painting on pure tea tree oil relieved nail fungus as effectively as 1 per cent clotrimazole.

The chemicals in tea tree oil have the unique property of mixing with sebaceous secretions to penetrate the top layers of skin, so they carry their antiseptic properties deeper than most emollient creams. This makes it a useful treatment for acne, furunculosis and boils.

Research continues into the effect of tea tree oil in MRSA infections.

It also has mild anaesthetic action and can be used on burns either directly or as a non-greasy cream.

The main topical uses are:

- Wounds – as an antiseptic
- Skin infections, such as acne vulgaris, boils and abscesses.
- Stings
- Thrush – oral and vaginal
- Athlete's foot/ringworm
- Minor burns and scalds including sunburn
- Fungal infections of the nails
- As a gargle for gum disease and sore throats

Unwanted effects

- Rarely reported skin reactions

Interactions with other herbs/drugs/vitamins

- None

Contraindications

- Known sensitivity to the plant or its derivatives

Recommended dosage

As a cream for skin infections

Diluted 1:5 with an inert carrier oil

1-5 drops in 200ml warm water

Lemon Balm ~ *Melissa officinalis*

Early scientific data reported the usefulness of melissa's anti-bacterial and anti-viral properties. The effect of dried extract on cold sores was examined in a double blind placebo-controlled randomised trial. Thirty-four patients applied balm cream topically four times daily against 32 placebo patients who used an emollient cream for the same length of time. After five days the treatment group showed significant differences relative to placebo. These were:

- A shorter healing period
- No spread of infection
- Rapid reduction in itching, tingling, burning and swelling
- A longer period until next attack

Lemon balm can also be taken internally and its effects as an anti-depressant are covered on page 52.

Main topical uses
- Cold sores (*Herpes labialis*)

Unwanted effects
- None

Interactions with other herbs/drugs/vitamins
- None

Contraindications
- None

Recommended dosage
Use as a cream twice daily
Or apply tincture of melissa with a cotton bud

Marigold ~ *Calendula officinalis*

This is a cottage garden favourite with healing and anti-inflammatory actions that have a special affinity for the skin. The flowers are used medicinally and are often made into an infusion or cream.

Anti-viral activity against HIV, rhinoviruses and vesicular stomatitis viruses has been noted. In addition calendula increased tumour latency, suppressed mammary tumour growth and enhanced lymphocyte proliferation in animal experiments.

Main topical uses
- Wounds
- Chapped skin/lips
- Skin inflammation

Unwanted effects
- Allergy to the plant

Interactions with other herbs/drugs/vitamins
- None

Contraindications
- Pregnancy and breastfeeding

Recommended dosage
Apply cream every two hours when a cold sore is erupting.
Or use diluted tincture to bathe the affected area.

13 | Menopause

Medicine is not only a science; it is also an art. It does not consist of compounding pills and plasters; it deals with the very processes of life, which must be understood before they may be guided.
~ Paracelsus (c1493-1541) *Die grosse Wundarznei*

The menopause marks that time in every woman's life when menstruation stops and she is no longer able to conceive and bear children naturally. It is really the date of her last menstrual period but has come to mean the transition lasting from several months to several years (known in the medical profession as the climacteric), sometimes also referred to as the peri-menopause. In the UK the average age for cessation of periods is 50 years 9 months.

This does not mark the end of sexuality or creativity. Indeed many women, freed from the limitations of monthly periods, contraception and pregnancy, find they feel more liberated and have more commitment and energy.

It is a natural condition for all women, not a disease process, and cannot be prevented or cured. Although some 75 per cent of women experience some symptoms at this stage in their lives it has been estimated that only 10 to 15 per cent seek medical attention.

Unfortunately, those who do have problems seem to be offered HRT or drugs only, without any discussion at all about what non-drug alternatives are available, what works best and for what particular symptoms. In my career I have prescribed HRT many times and continue to believe that for some women it is a suitable and appropriate treatment, enhancing their lives and removing symptoms that are difficult and very distressing.

But there are also many women for whom taking HRT would be an unjustifiable risk to their health, either because of a past history of thrombosis or other health problems that would be worsened by its administration (see later).

Many women who have experienced hormone-related cancers or who have a family history of them, for instance breast and ovarian cancers, may feel cautious about taking any hormonal therapies at all including hormonal contraceptives (the Pill) and HRT.

Women suffering or recovering from other cancers may feel apprehensive about taking additional hormones despite suffering from troublesome menopausal symptoms and would prefer to consider alternative remedies.

There are also a large number of women who have no other health problems but would like a more natural way to solve any symptoms that they may experience.

A survey of British women showed that 17 per cent of 393 post-menopausal women asked were currently receiving HRT, and 11 per cent had taken HRT but stopped because they were anxious about it or had suffered unwanted effects.

The average woman is postmenopausal for greater than one third of her life and with our ever-increasing lifespan this proportion is likely to increase. In the UK 20 per cent of the population, or approximately 12 million women, are aged over 50 years. There are many women who experience an artificially early menopause either due to surgery or radiotherapy for cancer treatment who will be post-menopausal for many more years than nature intended.

The good news is that many alternatives are available. In my experience they work very well for the majority of symptoms. Unfortunately there is, as yet, little except anecdotal evidence about long term effects on diseases such as heart disease.

The menopause may lead to a variety of unpleasant symptoms:

Acute

- Hot flushes
- Night sweats
- Insomnia
- Depression
- Anxiety symptoms
- Irritability

- Forgetfulness
- Difficulty in concentration
- Loss of confidence
- Palpitations

Intermediate

- Stress incontinence/urinary frequency/pain on passing urine
- Rising several times in the night to pass urine
- Dry skin and hair
- Dry vagina leading to inflammation, pain and even bleeding
- Painful intercourse
- Loss of interest in sex
- Aches and pains

Long-term

- Osteoporosis
- Changes in lipid metabolism, leading to ischaemic heart disease and strokes

Often support, advice and reassurance are all that are required but often, because of persistent or troublesome symptoms, patients are offered the following drugs:

A. Hypnotics, sedatives and tranquillisers, often benzodiazepines such as Oxazepam, Diazepam, and Chlordiazepoxide, although they have never been shown to relieve symptoms entirely caused by oestrogen deficiency.

B. Antidepressants – many women have only been offered anti-depressants as a non-hormonal alternative to HRT. Most are not depressed but it is now known that hot flushes cause physical discomfort, which affects quality of sleep in all ways: length of time slept, early waking and depth of sleep. Sleeplessness can lead to feelings of being out of control of domestic and work environments and loss of self-confidence. These symptoms are easily mistaken for depression if a thorough history, including a menstrual history, is not taken.

It is obvious that women suffering from depression will also experience menopausal symptoms but I feel that anti-depressants should be reserved for those women with classical symptoms of a depressive illness.

C. β-blockers are used to reduce the number of hot flushes. In my opinion they are not effective. They have also been used where anxiety is a troublesome feature of the menopause.

D. Clonidine was first reported to have beneficial effects on hot flushes in 1973. However, in other studies of longer duration, no benefits were found. It is still widely used.

E. Progesterone supplements by mouth or as a long-acting injection have been found to reduce hot flushes when compared to placebo. There may be an increased risk of osteoporosis with this treatment. Generally, it is rarely given without oestrogens.

F. 'Natural' progesterone creams are classed as cosmetics and not medicines and so have never been fully evaluated for safety and effectiveness. They are made with plant chemicals (sterols) found in herbs like Mexican yam. Most manufacturers are vague about the actual contents of these creams but they appear to vary widely in hormonal content. They are poorly absorbed through the skin, do not ease menopausal symptoms nor prevent osteoporosis and may even be carcinogenic.

G. Tibolone is a drug used to relieve hot flushes and prevent osteoporosis. It cannot be commenced until a year after the last menstrual period. After absorption it is changed within the body into two molecules with oestrogenic activity and one with progestagenic activity. It is not recommended for certain patients – those who have hormone dependent tumours such as breast or ovarian cancers; heart problems; disorders of the blood vessels around the brain or stroke; liver disease; or patients taking certain medications such as:

- Barbiturates
- Anticoagulants such as warfarin
- Rifampicin
- Carbamazepine
- Hydantoins

H. Hormone Replacement Treatment (HRT) – this relieves troublesome menopausal symptoms for a number of women. It is a combination of oestrogen and progesterone usually taken in a monthly cyclical pattern to mimic the natural menstrual cycle. HRT can be taken by mouth, applied as patches to the skin, or as an implant placed in the layer of fat just under the skin.

• Women treated with HRT had a significant improvement in symptoms when compared to a control group.

• HRT is known to reduce the osteoporosis risk in those one in four women at risk of fracture by 30 per cent from hip fracture and 50 per cent for spinal fracture.

• There are also beneficial effects on Alzheimer's disease and heart disease, though current recommendations are that it should not be prescribed on the basis of cardiovascular disease prevention only.

• Increasing evidence supports an association between HRT and a reduced risk of colorectal cancer.

• Localised vaginal symptoms can be treated with vaginal creams, tablets or pessaries. If the uterus is still present oestrogen should never be given on its own except in very small concentrations as this can cause the lining of the womb to be over-stimulated leading eventually to increased risk of uterine cancer. Cyclical progesterone (by mouth) should also be given.

Some of these treatments have unwanted effects:

A. The hypnotics, sedatives and tranquillisers are known to affect concentration, mood, sleep, digestion and other aspects of your health (see page 18).

B. Antidepressants. These are covered in detail on page 42.

C. The β-blocker group of drugs causes unwanted effects in 75 per cent of people. These are discussed in detail on page 22.

D. Clonidine is known to have the following unwanted effects:

- Low blood pressure
- Slow pulse
- Irregular heartbeat
- Drowsiness
- Constipation
- Impotence
- Disturbances in blood flow to hands and feet
- Changes in liver function
- Skin rashes
- Pain in the parotid (salivary) glands
- Depression
- Drying of nasal mucosa
- Reduced tears

E. Progesterone tablets/injections are known to have the following unwanted effects:

- Weight gain
- Irregular vaginal bleeding or absence of periods
- Headache
- Nervousness
- Abdominal pain or discomfort
- Changes in breast size and/or production of breast milk
- Sexual difficulties such as decreased sex drive, inability to reach orgasm
- Hair loss
- Varicose veins
- Skin rashes
- Increased risk of thrombosis
- Increased risk of osteoporosis
- Increased risk of breast cancer
- Worsening of following conditions: Diabetes mellitus, Depression, Migraine.

F. 'Natural' progesterone creams are known to have the following unwanted effects:
- Weight gain
- May lower immune response
- Fluid retention
- Allergy to components

G. Tibolone is known to have the following unwanted effects:
- Vaginal bleeding or spotting
- Change of body weight
- Dizziness
- Rash or itching
- Increased facial hair growth
- Headache and migraine
- Visual disturbances including blurred vision
- Nausea, indigestion
- Muscle pains

Although a definite relationship between the medication and problem has not been established, the following effects have also been reported:
- Uterine cancer
- Pulmonary and deep vein thrombosis
- Tibolone has caused worsening of the following conditions: Liver disorders, Renal disease, Epilepsy, Migraine, High blood cholesterol, Diabetes mellitus

H. HRT is known to have the following unwanted effects:
- Some women return to having regular menstrual periods. There are preparations that don't bring about menstruation but most of these should be commenced one year or so after the cessation of the usual monthly period.
- Weight gain or weight loss can occur. It is not possible to predict if either of these will occur.

- Some patients experience nausea, vomiting, abdominal cramps, bloating and jaundice. Using an implant or patch can often prevent this. There is a threefold increased risk of gallstone formation in women using HRT.

- Vaginal thrush, cystitis-like symptoms have been known to be persistent and troublesome.

- HRT can destroy vitamin B6 in the body, leading to depression, muscle cramps, dizziness and peripheral numbness. Some women who use HRT experience troublesome leg cramps especially at night.

- Skin pigmentation which may persist even after treatment is discontinued.

- Hair loss may occur on the scalp while body or facial hair may increase.

- Changes in the corneal curvature of the eye and intolerance to contact lenses are seen occasionally. There may be an increased risk of dry eye syndrome in HRT users.

- Many women notice an increase or diminution in sex drive. Unfortunately, as in the case of weight changes, it is difficult to predict what each individual woman will experience.

- Ankle swelling can occur.

- It has been reported that some women who take HRT notice breast tenderness, breast enlargement or milk secretion. It usually resolves when treatment is discontinued.

- Some women experience pre-menstrual syndrome feelings with mood changes, breast tenderness, bloating, etc, before a period (if applicable).

- Studies of women taking HRT have demonstrated an increased risk of venous thrombosis (blood clot in the veins of the body) threefold. This means that for every 1000 women treated there will be three cases of thrombosis – either deep vein thrombosis (in the deep veins of the legs) or pulmonary embolism (in the veins of the lungs) that would not otherwise have occurred.

- These studies have also shown an increased risk of stroke by up to 3.5 times. This risk is at its greatest during the first year of usage.

- Studies of women taking HRT have demonstrated an increased risk of ovarian cancer.

- There also appears to be an increased risk of endometrial (uterine) cancer. This amounts to 20 extra cases per 1000 women after five years of treatment.

- HRT gives an increased risk of breast cancer – data from 51 studies show that long-term oestrogen therapy increases risk of breast cancer slightly. A review of over 160,000 women both with and without breast cancer shows that there are two extra cases per 1000 women above those statistically expected to develop breast cancer in the group taking HRT for up to five years. There were three to nine extra cases in the group taking HRT for five to 10 years and there were five to 20 extra cases in the taking HRT for 15 or more years. This increased risk largely disappears within five years of stopping HRT. The risk is no different between those on combined treatment and oestrogen alone. Another difficulty encountered while taking HRT is that the density of breast tissue increases making interpretation of mammograms more difficult and early abnormalities harder to detect.

- However, in women who have breast cancer the risk of recurrence in the affected breast may be reduced by HRT although there may still be an increased risk in the previously unaffected breast.

- Women who have uterine fibroids will probably notice a gradual increase in their size over many months or years when taking HRT.

- Research shows that there is a general worsening of diabetic control and therefore higher risk of diabetic complications.

- There is conflicting evidence on the risk of heart disease. A large study found early harm and late benefits in women with coronary heart disease; the clinical trial documented more coronary events in the HRT group than in the placebo group. In countries where there is a low level of heart disease in women such as Italy, HRT did not protect women against coronary heart disease but increased their risk. Other trials reported benefits for patients with coronary artery disease.

- HRT has been shown to produce worsening of the following conditions: Cancers of breast and womb; Liver disease; Kidney disease;

Migraine; Fibrocystic disease of the breast; Otosclerosis; Asthma; Multiple sclerosis; Systemic lupus erythematosis; Porphyria; Endometriosis; Epilepsy; Melanoma, Hypertension.

Helpful lifestyle changes

These can make a marked difference to some short term and more long-term problems experienced in the menopause. Many, but not all, of these recommendations are nutritionally based. You will see that some foods come under two or three different categories because they are beneficial to more than one aspect of your metabolism and health.

Some 20-21 minerals, 13 vitamins, eight to 10 amino acids and two essential fatty acids have, so far, been identified as necessary for normal bodily function and good health. Many are essential – in biological terms this means that we cannot manufacture them in our bodies, but must eat and assimilate them.

Smoking

Stopping smoking (both active and passive) is the single most important thing you can do to improve your long-term health and prevent illnesses such as heart disease.

Exercise

Physical activity is also important. More than 100 studies show the benefits of regular weight-bearing exercise on bone strength and on the heart. Exercise can slow age related mental decline and can reduce the risk of Alzheimer's disease. Exercise also cuts the risk of obesity, heart disease, diabetes mellitus and stroke.

You don't have to pump iron at the gym – a regular brisk walk around the block, lasting 30 minutes, at least three times a week is just as beneficial, though the more exercise taken within sensible limits, the greater the effect. Excess exercise can be as harmful as none. Those who train too intensively may be at risk of low body mass and absent menstruation (if relevant) leading to increased risk of osteoporosis.

You may prefer a more sociable activity like badminton, bowls, golf or line dancing, but even 30 minutes of strenuous gardening or housework will provide some health benefits.

Sex

An active sex life is good for you! It stimulates hormone production, including the brain chemicals or endorphins that make us feel good; relieves tension and makes us feel calmer. In a huge research project conducted in San Francisco 55,000 people were asked about their health and their sex lives. Researchers concluded that those who had a satisfying sex life were, on the whole, healthier than those who did not.

Diet

Ensure that your diet is balanced, rich in natural phyto-oestrogens, and contains sufficient vitamins, minerals and essential fatty acids. Always start the day with breakfast and eat three proper meals per day. Plan your menu for the week so that you are not tempted to buy convenience foods. Always buy the best that you can afford. Avoid processed foods that are high in salt, low in vitamins and high in additives.

If possible, shop twice weekly for fresh vegetables and fruit.

The following have special relevance during the menopause but make sure that your diet contains all the necessary micronutrients.

In a small number of clinical trials increasing consumption of soya products reduced the severity but not the frequency of hot flushes. It makes sense, therefore, to consume foods high in natural plant oestrogens every day such as soya products (soya flour, soya milk, soya beans, tofu) peanuts and other leguminous vegetables (peas, red kidney beans, etc), fennel, celery, pomegranates, parsley, and linseed. Phyto-oestrogens are also found in grains such as rye, wheat and oats.

A review study of research into soya in the diet showed a protective role against cancer in more than a half of animal studies.

In a two-year case-controlled study of women, aged 30-84, in Perth, Australia, those with a high intake of plant oestrogens had a significantly lower risk of contracting breast cancer. Epidemiological studies confirm that those women who live where there is a large intake of plant oestrogens, usually from a soya rich diet, have lower frequency of menopausal symptoms and a lower rate of breast cancer.

Vitamin E (1000mg per day)

Tests dramatically support its use for hot flushes. It also helps to calm anxiety and ease vaginal dryness (200-800mg/day). Inserting a vitamin E capsule into the vagina can be helpful for severe vaginal dryness. Patients taking 800-1000mg per day had fewer menopausal symptoms.

Vitamin E supplements have also been associated with a reduced risk of heart disease.

Vitamin E is found naturally in:

- Nuts and seeds: Sunflower seeds; Walnuts; Almonds; Hazelnuts; Peanuts (not salted); Brazil nuts; Pecans.

- Legumes; Soya beans; Lima beans.

- Brans; Wheat bran; Wheat germ; Rice bran.

Vitamin C (1000mg per day)
This is found in most fresh fruit and vegetables especially citrus fruits, kiwi fruit and strawberries. For an intake of this amount you may need to take a supplement. Vitamin C can be taken in combination with vitamin E which also relieved flushes, cramps, etc. Only a few unwanted effects were experienced but some patients had diarrhoea, which can be caused by high levels of vitamin C.

Vitamin C has many beneficial effects, reducing the blood's tendency to clot, acting as an antioxidant, reducing levels of LDL cholesterol, having anti-cancer properties and protecting against heart disease.

Bioflavonoids
Certain bioflavonoids (quercetin and its derivatives) may have an oestrogenic effect and may also have a role in preventing stroke. Quercetin is found in garlic, onions, most fruits, vegetables and grains. Black tea and rooibosch (redbush) tea are other sources.

Vitamin D
This can be made in the skin during exposure to sunlight; it is needed for adequate absorption of calcium. If your diet is high in calcium – fish, eggs, dried fruit, pulses – consider exposing your skin to regular small periods (20 minutes) of sunlight without using a sunscreen, to achieve maximum absorption and utilisation of the mineral.

There is no doubt that sunlight is the best source of vitamin D and people who cover up all the time have lower levels of this essential vitamin. Skin pigmentation also greatly reduces its production. Some foods are high in vitamin D such as eggs, fortified cereals like *Rice Crispies*, fish liver oil and oily fish such as mackerel and salmon. If you are unable to sunbathe in the summer months, (and in winter where sunlight levels are lower), then supplement your diet with vitamin D (10μg per day). You will find most vitamins are now sold in milligrams (mg) or micrograms (μg). Vitamin D used to be measured in iu (international units), 1μg vitamin D = 40iu. This is left over from the days when the chemical structure of these micronutrients was unknown and they were measured in terms of biological activity. As their structures were discovered they could be measured in terms of their weight and iu became obsolete. However you may see values in either measurement. 10μg vitamin D would be equivalent to 400iu.

B Complex Vitamins
These reduce fluid retention and contribute to a healthy thyroid, therefore combating fatigue, fluid retention, etc. The tablet you choose should contain at least 25-50mg vitamin B6, 2.0μg vitamin B12 and 300μg folic acid (vitamin B9). B vitamins are found naturally in unrefined cereals, green leafy vegetables, liver and offal and wholewheat.

Vitamin A
Take care not to consume too much vitamin A. Over 20 years, 120,000 American nurses not taking HRT were studied and it was concluded that an intake over 2000μg vitamin A per day lead to an increased risk of osteoporotic fracture by 50 per cent. The ideal supplement should contain 1000μg of vitamin A. It is found naturally in fish liver oils, liver, carrots, dark green leafy vegetables and eggs.

Calcium, Magnesium, Vitamin D and Phosphorus
These minerals and vitamin D are the best-known minerals and vitamins needed to help prevent osteoporosis. Risk factors for osteoporosis are:

• Low birth weight denoting poor intra-uterine nutrition
• Poor nutrition in childhood and adolescence
• Lack of physical activity in childhood and adolescence
• Smoking
• Excess alcohol
• Excess coffee

- Lack of physical activity
- Low body weight (Body Mass Index <20)
- Poor nutrition including anorexia nervosa
- Drinks high in phosphoric and citric acid such as cola drinks
- Premature menopause
- Hysterectomy under 45 years, even if ovaries remain
- Medically/surgically induced menopause
- Steroid therapy (for more than six months)
- Hyperthyroidism
- Cystic fibrosis
- Coeliac disease
- Organ transplant with immunosuppressive therapy
- Previous fracture
- Maternal fracture

Osteoporosis is symptom free unless a fracture occurs. It is a debilitating disease with severe weakening of the bones. Fractures readily occur, and broken wrists and collapsed spinal vertebrae are painful and disfiguring. However the most devastating injury is hip fracture – one in four women and one in six men will suffer from this.

By age 70, 50 per cent of women sustain a hip fracture, and often the patient never walks again, losing their independence. In 1998 there were 70,000 hip fractures, costing the NHS £942 million. Tragically, during the period of disability many people's health can deteriorate markedly sometimes even terminally.

In the UK hip fracture is associated with 14,000 deaths per year. Worldwide some 200 million people suffer from osteoporosis.

Calcium

Calcium is the best-known mineral with the ability to ward off osteoporosis. If your intake is high in teenage years you may have up to 40 per cent lower risk of fracture in later life. In most people maximum bone strength occurs at about 35 years old. After that there is a gradual decrease in mineral density and no matter how much calcium you eat this will not change substantially. The ideal is to take in sufficient calcium to slow the losses and ward off fractures.

How much calcium do you need daily to keep your bones healthy? Postmenopausal women probably get full bone protection from 900-1000mg of calcium per day.

In a study reported in 1997 subjects were given either placebo or calcium 500mg + vitamin D3, 400iu daily for three years. The supplement reduced the incidence of spinal fractures in post-menopausal women by half (59 per cent v 12.9 per cent).

Surprisingly the best sources of calcium seem to be non-dairy such as fish (including canned fish with bones), peanuts, sesame seeds, sunflower seeds, hard water, kale, broccoli and other green vegetables. Possibly the high phosphate content in milk prevents full absorption of its calcium content.

In a recent study in the USA women who drank two pints of milk per day doubled their risk of hip fracture! This was backed up by a Norwegian study which concluded that women who drank the most milk suffered the most fractures.

Beverages high in phosphoric acid such as cola drinks deplete the body of calcium. Eating a low fat diet may have a bad effect on bone strength because fat is needed to absorb calcium.

Magnesium

You should always take a magnesium supplement if you are going to take calcium in a 2:1 ratio of calcium to magnesium. This is needed for the production and maintenance of healthy bone and muscles. It is found naturally in nuts, grains, beans, dark green vegetables, fish and meat. People taking diuretics (water tablets) such as Bendrofluazide and Frusemide, and laxatives are most likely to be deficient. Deficiency is also more common in diabetic patients, alcoholics and patients with heart problems. The daily recommended dose is 250-300mg.

Manganese

Bones benefit from a regular intake of manganese. In laboratory studies animals deprived of this mineral developed osteoporosis. Women with osteoporosis have been found to have about one third less manganese in their blood than healthy women.

One of the richest sources of this mineral is pineapple. It is also found in oatmeal, nuts, cereals, beans, whole wheat, spinach and tea. The recommended dose is 5-20mg daily. Do not be tempted to take more than this, as excessive intake has been associated with forms of dementia and psychiatric symptoms. Patients with liver disorders should not supplement with manganese, as they cannot excrete any excess.

Selenium

Eat a variety of nuts regularly – they are high in fibre, mono-unsaturated fats and selenium (you need 200mcg of selenium daily), which is necessary to maintain normal hormone function and may have a role in the prevention of cancer. They are also thought to promote a healthy heart and encourage normal function of the thyroid gland. Just eating a few every day will be beneficial, but avoid salted nuts.

Boron

Foods high in the mineral boron can boost oestrogen levels naturally. Boron is found in fruit (other than citrus fruits) especially apples, pears, grapes, dates, raisins and peaches, legumes especially soya beans, nuts especially almonds, peanuts, hazelnuts, vegetables and honey. Supplements should not exceed 3mg per day.

Salt

Too much salt reduces bone density. Try to cut added salt out of your diet by reducing consumption of such foods as salted peanuts, bacon, chips, snack foods and reduce the amount you use in cooking. If you like a lot of salt on your food, try substituting one of the low salt products available on the market, such as LoSalt, for your usual table salt. Elderly women in New Zealand were put on a low salt diet then switched to a high salt diet. They ate the same amount of calcium on both. On the high salt diet 30 per cent more calcium was lost.

Fats and Oils

In general reduce the amount of fat and oil in your diet but note that some fats and oils are beneficial to health while others are harmful.

Some women have almost developed a phobia about eating fats but Professor Walter Willett of Harvard Medical School found no correlation between fat intake and breast cancer. Women on low fat diets had just as much chance of developing this type of cancer than those on a high fat diet. It has been known for at least 20 years that lowering fat intake and cholesterol intake does not appear to make much difference to total plasma concentrations of cholesterol.

Many doctors now believe that a low fat diet contributes to osteoporosis by preventing absorption of calcium and other important minerals. However, it is important to eat sufficient of the right sorts of fats:

- Oil of evening primrose 1000mg, hemp seed oil 1000mg or flaxseed oil 1000mg help to control oestrogen production. A supplement of any can help to maintain hormone levels or you can add linseeds (flaxseeds) to your diet. Evening primrose oil has been shown to kill cancer cells without harming normal cells in tissue cultures.

- Increase your intake of mono-unsaturates, found in virgin olive oils and nuts.

- Increase your intake of oily fish (mackerel, salmon, and sardines) to 35g or fish oils to 1000mg, two to five times per week. This has numerous benefits, including protection against heart attack and stroke by as much as 53 per cent. Even moderate consumption, ie once a week, can reduce the risk by 2 per cent. The oils found in fish also promote production of natural anti-inflammatory agents within the body. These protect joints against the onset of osteoarthritis. Other studies show that fish oils slow down the growth of tumours.

- Avoid saturated or animal fats. High intakes have been linked to heart disease and cancer formation, probably because they promote inflammation in the body. Aim to have no more than 5 per cent of your calories as saturated fats.

- Avoid trans fatty acids – these come from partially hydrogenated vegetable oils and are associated with cancer formation. They are found in margarine, biscuits and chocolates, and particularly foods consumed by vegetarians and those who wish to avoid cholesterol and saturated fats.

The incidence of heart disease usually rises after the menopause. This is widely believed to be due to adverse changes in lipid and lipoprotein metabolism due to low oestrogen levels. These changes in fats in the blood increase the risk of heart disease.

Weight

If you are overweight take steps to reduce your weight to within the normal range for your age. Try to keep your body mass index (BMI) between 20 and 25. This is calculated by:

$$BMI = \frac{Weight\ in\ kg}{Height\ in\ metres^2}$$

Being overweight increases your risk of heart disease, diabetes and even cancer. However, being underweight increases the risk of osteoporosis, as does dieting for long periods. Your practice nurse or nurse practitioner should be able to advise you.

Researchers at the University of California found that although older women were often advised to lose significant amounts of weight for health reasons, this could lead to a loss in bone density. Don't crash diet. If your diet is already healthy and you have cut down on saturated fats (not essential fatty acids), try reducing carbohydrate intake (sugar, bread and pasta) or, better still, increase the amount of exercise that you take. Remember that this is not a lifestyle change for a few weeks but a change for the rest of your life.

Also make sure that you eat five helpings of fresh fruit or vegetables per day excluding potatoes. Try to eat half of these raw.

Garlic

Garlic taken over several months has been shown to reduce blood cholesterol by as much as 15 per cent and reduce risk of heart attack by 30 per cent. Recent research links breast cancer to high cholesterol. Just taking half a clove of garlic daily has been shown to reduce blood stickiness, and tablets containing 10mg allicin lowered triglycerides and bad LDL cholesterol by 15 per cent.

Natural garlic is far superior to capsules in this respect because deodorised products do not contain all the active components and their action is less beneficial. Cooking does not destroy garlic's action.

Garlic is also known to have anti-cancer, anti-inflammatory and anti-ageing effects.

Canned drinks

Avoid canned drinks high in phosphoric acid or citric acid as these remove calcium from the body and makes osteoporosis more likely. Citric acid is also added to fruit drinks, fruit yoghurt and fruit puddings.

Artificial sweeteners

Avoid all artificial sweeteners. They are synthetic chemicals and their safety is in doubt. Unfortunately, because they are classed as foods and not drugs, there is no post-marketing surveillance to assess their safety. Some are banned in other countries because of possible risks to health. Aspartame (E951), Acesulfame–K, Saccharin (E954) and Thaumatin are the ones you are most likely to encounter.

Coffee and tea

Cutting out tea and coffee may help to reduce hot flushes. They tend to be vasodilators and make you flush more easily and more often.

Otherwise drinking up to three cups of coffee a day seems safe. Recent research shows that moderate caffeine intake is not detrimental to bone strength, but more than this may cause leaching of calcium from the bones. A recent study of 84,000 middle-aged women found that those who drank more than four cups of coffee per day were approximately three times more likely to suffer hip fractures than those who drank little or no caffeine. Tea exhibited no adverse effects.

Alcohol

Some women notice an increase in hot flushes when they drink alcohol. When acute flushes have ceased, a regular intake of alcohol – that is one to two measures daily – can boost oestrogen levels by 10-20 per cent. Research at the University of Pittsburgh USA, found that alcohol boosts oestrogen possibly by stimulating an enzyme in the liver that converts androgens to oestradiol.

Beer and bourbon that is derived from corn had slightly greater action; even de-ethanolized bourbon was biologically active. Hops – a constituent of beers – contain natural oestrogens (see page 46). A regular small intake of alcohol has long been known to have a cardio-protective effect, possibly because it also has a beneficial effect on cholesterol levels, is an anti-coagulant and contains anti-oxidants. It reduces heart attacks by 40 per cent.

However larger intakes are well known to have a detrimental effect on many aspects of health. Women who consume large amounts of alcohol regularly may increase their risk of illness by 45-50 per cent, according to an American study. Be sure to reduce the one to two unit daily recommended amount if you are of small height or build. These recommendations are based on an average 70kg woman. If you are smaller you will have a smaller liver and the amount you take should be correspondingly less.

Acidophilus

Acidophilus are beneficial bacteria and should be consumed regularly. As well as maintaining the balance of normal bacteria in the colon they help to combat any tendency to soreness in the vaginal area that may occur with ageing. In a study carried out by Dr Eileen Hilton at the Long Island Medical Centre in New York a group of women with recurrent vaginitis were divided into two groups. The first ate a cup of 'live' yoghurt daily; the second did not. The first group had a threefold lower incidence of vaginal soreness and pain during sex than the control group. If you don't like yoghurt, acidophilus is available as a capsule.

Depression

If you suffer from depression it may be because lower levels of plasma oestrogen make less tryptophan available for conversion to serotonin (a mood-regulating hormone naturally present in the brain). Some foods are higher in this essential amino acid (poultry, fish, bananas, dried dates, and peanuts). Eating a good portion of one or more of these per day may ease symptoms of depression. Calcium and magnesium ease anxiety (calcium 1-1.5g daily in a 2:1 ratio with magnesium).

Coenzyme Q10

Think prevention when it comes to breast cancer. Coenzyme Q10 (90-1200mg daily) together with antioxidants and essential fatty acids have been successful in the treatment and secondary prevention of breast cancer.

If symptoms persist and are troublesome there are several herbs with long track records of treating menopausal symptoms successfully and easing the transition into a post-menopausal state.

In many cases it is not known precisely how a particular herb works. It has been noted for centuries that some work better for some women than others. I have included the herbs in the order which, in my experience, they seem to be effective for most women. If one does not seem to have a beneficial effect try adding another. I do not recommend taking more than three at a time.

A few herbs are most useful for particular problems such as heavy periods. I have included these toward the end of this chapter.

Refer to chapters 1 and 2 for treatment of problems such as anxiety and depression.

Herbs work well. They contain many different phyto-chemicals which are responsible for their action. Some regulate hormones, some balance hormone levels and others reduce other unwanted symptoms of the menopause such as hot flushes. In isolation I doubt that the individual chemicals would be as well tolerated or effective at reducing unpleasant effects of the menopause.

Black Cohosh ~ *Cimicifuga racemosa*

Black cohosh was used in traditional Native American medicine to treat female problems like menstrual cramps and menopausal symptoms. The aerial parts of the plant are used medicinally.

It is one of the most thoroughly researched herbs for the treatment of menopausal symptom especially in Germany. It does not contain oestrogen.

A recent study involving 629 women favourably compared its ability to relieve symptoms of the menopause with Premarin (HRT). Black cohosh reduced menopausal symptoms in 80 per cent of women within six weeks. There was one big difference however – there were scarcely any unwanted effects especially in terms of weight gain, risk of thrombosis, etc.

Studies show that the herb contains natural compounds that bind to oestrogen receptors and cause a selective reduction in the level of luteinising hormone produced by the pituitary gland.

In animal studies it has been found to inhibit the proliferation of breast cancer cells. This effect was weakened if oestrogens were given at the same time; conversely there was an increase in growth inhibition of cancer cells when it was used alongside Tamoxifen. This suggests that the beneficial effects of Tamoxifen for women with breast cancer are enhanced by black cohosh. More research needs to be done to see if this has a similar effect in women, but the evidence is very encouraging.

There are also positive findings in terms of prevention of heart disease, especially heart attacks and osteoporosis in postmenopausal women.

In addition it has a marked anti-hypertensive effect for some people.

Uses

- Menopausal symptoms
- Joint muscle, nerve pain and muscular cramps

Unwanted effects

- Gastrointestinal discomfort
- Headache
- Low blood pressure
- Weight changes
- Myalgia/muscle pains

Interactions with other herbs

- Sedative herbs

Interactions with other drugs

- Sedative and tranquillising drugs

Contraindications

- Pregnancy and breastfeeding
- Cancer of breast

Recommended dosage

Capsules or tablets	200–400mg daily
Tincture	0.4–2ml daily
Fluid extract	0.2ml daily

Mexican Yam ~ *Dioscorea villosa*

The root of this plant aids generalised menopausal symptoms. It does not contain oestrogens or any other hormones as is widely, but mistakenly, believed. This medical myth has probably arisen from the fact that in 1956 Japanese researchers discovered glycoside saponins in several varieties of Mexican yams. Later steroidal saponins, most notably diosgenin, were derived from these tubers. They were converted in the laboratory to progesterone and other hormones such as androgens, oestrogens and corticosteroids. At one time *Dioscorea villosa* was the only source of raw material available for contraceptive pill manufacture.

Our bodies cannot produce progesterone or dihydroepiandrosterone from *Dioscorea*, but the diosgenin found in it can mimic the effects of oestrogen, thus helping to reduce symptoms due to oestrogen deficiency that arise in the menopause.

Uses
- Menopausal symptoms

Unwanted effects
- None

Interactions with other herbs
- None

Interactions with other drugs
- None

Contraindications
- None

Recommended dosage:
Capsules or tablets   up to 4g daily
Tinctures   up to 15ml daily

Red Clover Flowers ~ *Trifolium pratense*

In 1990 a study showed that women who consumed food and drink high in natural oestrogens and red clover supplements experienced the same changes in the lining of the vagina as women taking HRT.

There has been considerable research into red clover plants – however, as this is an important forage plant for cattle it has been conducted with agricultural rather than medicinal benefits in mind. It is difficult to ascertain whether some of the research has been done on red clover plants or red clover flowers.

Its main use in current practice is to help to reduce the acute symptoms of the menopause. Its effectiveness comes from its high level of isoflavones (1 to 2.5 per cent), which helps to promote normal oestrogen levels and occupy oestrogen receptor sites as an alternative to oestrogen.

Red clover has been used since the time of Hippocrates. It is traditionally considered to have anti-cancer properties and has been widely used 'for reduction of tumours and hard swellings' by the physicians of the ancient world.

Uses

- Menopausal symptoms

Unwanted effects

- None

Interactions with other herbs

- None

Interactions with other drugs

- Warfarin and other anti-coagulants

Contraindications

- Oestrogen dependent cancers such as breast, ovary, womb
- Pregnancy and breastfeeding
- Tendency to bleed

Recommended dosage

Infusion	up to 10g daily
Capsules or tablets	up to 5g daily
Tincture	up to 20ml daily

Fenugreek ~ *Trigonella foenum-graecum*

The seeds of this plant are used medicinally. They contain diosgenin and tigogenin which can act as a substitute for oestrogen when the amount in the body diminishes during the menopause. It can also help to regulate blood sugar and lower cholesterol levels. The seeds encourage normal bowel movements. Fenugreek has a powerful curry flavour that is hard to disguise and may not be to everyone's taste. It is more palatable if taken as a capsule or tablet.

Uses

- Menopausal symptoms
- Regulation of blood sugar
- Lowering of cholesterol levels
- Constipation

Unwanted effects

- None

Interactions with other herbs

- None

Interactions with other drugs

- There is some evidence that the absorption of other drugs may be delayed.

Contraindications

- Pregnancy and breastfeeding
- Diabetes mellitus (may lower blood sugar)

Recommended dosage

Seeds   up to 2 cupfuls daily
Capsules   up to 5g daily
Tincture   up to 15ml daily

Raspberry Leaf ~ *Rubus ideus*

Raspberry leaf, as its name suggests, is the leaf of the domestic raspberry plant. It is therefore easily found in most kitchen gardens – a by-product, in fact, of your raspberry canes!

It has a particular affinity for the female reproductive tract. In country districts it remains a tonic to drink in the latter stages of pregnancy to prepare the system for labour. Raspberry leaf normalises uterine muscle tone and buffers the effects of abnormal hormone levels. It is particularly useful in the peri-menopause where irregular heavy periods are a problem.

Uses

• Heavy periods (menorrhagia) in the peri-menopause

Unwanted effects

• None

Interactions with other herbs

• None

Interactions with other drugs

• Absorption of other drugs may be delayed

Contraindications

• None

Recommended dosage
All to be taken three times a day
Dried herb as an infusion   5–10ml
Infusion   12– 24g daily
Liquid extract 1:1 in 25% alcohol   12–24ml daily

Liquorice Root ~ *Glycyrrhiza glabra*

This plant is mentioned in detail in chapter 7 as a treatment for digestive upset. It is well known for its oestrogenic activity. It is also known to be anti-inflammatory and anti-viral. At times of high stress liquorice is particularly useful because it supports the adrenal glands and controls production of stress hormones, as well as promoting natural production of sex hormones by the adrenals after the menopause. In China it is called the 'great detoxifier' and is thought to drive poisons from the system.

Although it has been claimed that liquorice gives unwanted effects – especially electrolyte imbalance – and can be toxic, whole liquorice root has never been shown to cause toxicity and I can find no evidence of the whole herb causing these problems. Highly concentrated liquorice extracts, such as liquorice-containing laxatives and carbenoxelone sodium-containing ulcer medications, do exhibit these unwanted effects.

Liquorice is recorded as a cancer treatment in many countries.

On its own liquorice is mildly laxative. Best results are obtained when liquorice is combined with other herbs.

When used medicinally remember that any intake of liquorice confectionery should be taken into account when calculating the dosage.

Uses

- Menopause
- Inflammatory conditions
- High blood cholesterol
- As a tonic stimulant for the adrenal glands. It is very useful if you are under stress.

Chinese Angelica ~ *Angelica sinensis*

This is one of two Chinese herbs that I sometimes recommend to patients during the menopause. It is also known as Dong Quai or Women's Ginseng. This rhizome has a long history of use in Asia for menstrual and menopausal problems where it is prescribed as the principal women's tonic herb.

Like many other 'women's herbs' it does not contain hormones but may increase circulation and blood supply to the body generally and to the pelvic organs in particular. This results in more energy, increasing vaginal tone and optimising the capability to produce the correct balance of hormones naturally. It is unlikely to improve hot flushes.

Main uses
- Menopausal debility

Unwanted effects
- None

Interactions with other herbs
- None

Interactions with other drugs
- Aspirin
- Warfarin
- Heparin
- Other anticoagulants

Contraindications
- Pregnancy and breastfeeding
- Acute viral illnesses
- Menorrhagia (heavy periods)
- Any condition that could lead to a tendency to bleed easily

Recommended dosage

Capsules or tablets	up to 5g daily
Tincture (diluted 1:3)	up to 15ml daily

Schizandra ~ *Schizandra chinensis*

This is another Chinese tonic herb. It is the fruit of an aromatic vine and has a reputation as a tonic and restorative for both sexes through its tonic effect on the liver and also on the reproductive organs. I have found it to have beneficial effects on the vaginal mucosa, improving lubrication and preventing dryness and painful sexual intercourse even where HRT has failed. It is most effective if combined with other herbs (see above).

Main uses
- Vaginal dryness
- Loss of libido

Unwanted effects
- Large doses may cause heartburn

Interactions with other herbs
- None

Interactions with other drugs
- None

Contraindications
- None

Recommended dosage
Decoction   up to 5g berries daily
Tincture   1ml three times daily

Hops ~ *Humulus lupulus*

This useful herb can be used during the menopause for anxiety and panic attacks. It is known to contain oestrogens as well as volatile oils and resin. Because hops also contain the bitter principle they have a beneficial effect on the gastro-intestinal tract. However, the bitter taste makes them unacceptable to some people. Hops have already been discussed on page 63 as a treatment for insomnia.

Main uses

- Anxiety
- Irritable bowel syndrome

Motherwort ~ *Leonurus cardiaca*

Motherwort is a member of the *Labiatae* family which includes mint and thyme. The leaves are used medicinally. The common name motherwort suggests a long association between this herb and women. It is particularly useful for menopausal symptoms such as anxiety, mood changes and palpitations.

Motherwort is used in almost all native medicinal pharmacopoeiae. It can be taken as a sedative and is very good for treating panic attacks and palpitations, having a generally soothing effect on the heart. It is antispasmodic and helps relaxation without causing sleepiness.

It has been discussed as a treatment for anxiety on page 31.

Uses

- Panic attacks, especially if accompanied with palpitations.
- Anxiety
- Antispasmodic

St John's Wort ~ *Hypericum perforatum*

The Knights of St John used it on the battlefields of the Crusades to promote the healing of wounds. Comparatively recently it has been found useful for treating depression and mood changes and is the medicine chosen by many German doctors to treat nervous problems.

St John's wort is a valuable herb in the menopause. It helps to reduce hot flushes and mood swings and possibly improves sleep. It works best if combined with other menopause herbs. It has been dealt with in detail on page 47.

Uses
- Menopausal problems, including hot flushes, anxiety, tension and depression.

Sage ~ *Salvia officinalis*

This is a well-known everyday herb which many women will already have growing in their gardens. It is excellent where there is excessive night sweating especially during the menopause, and can also reduce the number of hot flushes experienced during the day. Sage has a very strong characteristic flavour that is difficult to disguise and large doses are often required to be effective. This may make it unacceptable to some women.

Uses
- Menopausal night sweats
- Hot flushes

Unwanted effects
- None

Interactions with other herbs
- None

Interactions with other drugs
- None

Contraindications

- Haematuria (blood in the urine)
- Pregnancy
- Epilepsy

Recommended dosage

Average dose	1-3g daily
Infusion	15-30ml daily
Tincture 1:10 in 45% alcohol	6-12ml daily

Chasteberry/Monk's Pepper ~ *Vitex agnus castus*

This herb is known to have an effect on the anterior pituitary gland, encouraging normal levels of the stimulating hormones produced there. It is very useful for PMS and menopausal patients. Studies show that it increases luteinising hormone production, shifting the ratio of oestrogen to progestagen and thus addressing a corpus luteum hormone effect. It is therefore useful in treating menstrual disorders caused by a corpus luteum deficiency. It is licensed in Germany for menopausal symptoms. See chapter 14 for more information.

Uses

- Menopausal symptons

14 | Pre-Menstrual Syndrome (PMS) and Fibrocystic Disease of the Breasts

Her voice was ever soft, gentle and low, an excellent thing in woman
~ Shakespeare *King Lear* (Act 5, Scene 3)

Premenstrual syndrome is defined as physical and psychological symptoms occurring regularly during the luteal phase (second half) of the menstrual cycle. This phase occurs between ovulation and menstruation, ie between days 14 to 28 in a regular 28-day menstrual cycle. Symptoms vary in type and severity between different women and also between different cycles. What defines the condition is its recurring nature and the total resolution of symptoms at the beginning of a period. These symptoms are often collectively referred to as Pre-menstrual Tension (PMT).

Traditional wisdom has always equated PMS with hormonal imbalance but, to date, research has failed to demonstrate any consistent hormonal deficiency or excess and there may be complex patho-physiology at work. This includes possible deficiencies in vitamins and minerals.

The majority of menstruating women experience some symptoms before their period. It is estimated that five to 10 per cent of them have symptoms of sufficient severity to interfere with their job and/or personal life.

Several other health problems also show a pre-menstrual exacerbation. These include migraine, epilepsy, asthma, but it is not suggested that these be treated as PMS.

In women who have undergone hysterectomy but retained their ovaries, symptoms of PMS may still occur cyclically although periods will be absent.

Fibrocystic breast disease is a condition where breasts become tender, swollen painful and lumpy. It is usually worse in the time leading up to a period. Many of the measures listed below to improve PMS will also ease fibrocystic breast disease.

Typical symptoms include:

- Psychological problems – these are the commonest symptoms and may include irritability, depression, aggression, anxiety, tearfulness, fatigue, clumsiness, sleep disorders, loss of sex drive, and poor concentration.
- Breast problems – most predominantly pain, but swollen breasts may occur.
- Skin problems – flushing and sweating may occur. Acne may be a problem or pre-existing acne may flare up. Other skin conditions may also worsen temporarily.
- Gynaecological problems – mostly pelvic pain or a feeling of dragging or discomfort.
- Gastrointestinal symptoms are not as frequent but include abdominal pains, bloating, nausea and anorexia.
- Other problems such as joint stiffness and headache may occur.

There are several pharmaceutical therapies widely used for PMS. These include the following:

A .Bromocrytpine – the primary use of this drug is to treat tumours of the pituitary but it has also been used to treat premenstrual syndrome.

B. Diuretics – used to reduce the fluid retained before a period. This extra fluid is thought to lead to headaches, irritability, abdominal discomfort and breast tenderness.

C. Progesterones – these are the most commonly prescribed treatment for PMS in the UK and USA. The theory is that symptoms are caused by low progesterone levels in the second half of the cycle. An analysis of more than eight randomised trials does not support its use, except perhaps in the management of cyclical breast pain. In a meta-analysis of 14 randomised controlled trials involving 900 women, no significant evidence was found to support the use of progesterone in PMS.

D. Combined Oral Contraceptive Pill – this suppresses ovulation and in most women this will suppress symptoms too. Some women experience a resurgence of problems in the pill-free week. A possible solution is to take three packs consecutively, leaving only four or so weeks in the year where this would be a problem. This is only, in my opinion, a satisfactory alternative in women who wish to use the Pill as a contraceptive and should obviously be avoided in women with a history or family history of hormone related cancer.

E. Continuous oestrogen therapy is commonly used in the form of transdermal HRT – this is a skin patch that allows oestrogen to be absorbed into the body. Oestrogen is not licensed for PMS and is not a suitable choice for women with oestrogen dependent cancers. It will always be necessary to give progesterone from day 14 of the cycle to prevent abnormal proliferation of the lining and the womb and avoid development of uterine cancer. Progesterone can be given by mouth, vaginal application or in an intra-uterine system.

F. Gondotrophin releasing hormone analogues – such as Danazol. This is another drug method of suppressing ovulation which can be effective.

G. Antidepressants – a recent review of 20 medical studies concluded that selective serotonin reuptake inhibitors (SSRI) anti-depressants like Fluoxetine are effective in treating severe cases of PMS. This improved some of the physical symptoms of severe premenstrual syndrome as well as the psychological effects. It also mentioned that two and a half times more patients on SSRIs stopped their drugs due to unwanted effects than in the control group and those patients on other types of anti-depressants. These drugs don't address the fundamental problem of PMS, which is multifactorial. As the researchers say, the benefits could be a result of improved mood.

H. Anxiolytics are used when anxiety symptoms predominate. They have no specific use in PMS and do not address causative factors.

Sometimes unwanted effects of these drugs can be worse than the illness.

A. Unwanted effects of Bromocriptine include:

- Low blood pressure, which may be associated with falls. Patients on therapy for high blood pressure must be carefully watched if they take this medication. Dizziness and vomiting have also been experienced.

- Headache and drowsiness.
- Effects on the gut – gastro-intestinal bleeding has been reported. Nausea is the commonest unwanted effect.
- Effects on mood. Patients with a history of mental disorder or severe heart disease have exhibited severe psychiatric disturbance.
- Effects on the circulation. Pallor of the extremities, especially in patients with pre-existing circulation problems.
- Some patients have developed fluid around the lungs.
- Retroperitoneal fibrosis has been observed in patients on long-term treatment.
- Severe unwanted effects are rare, but include high blood pressure, stroke, mental disorders and seizures.

B. Unwanted effects of diuretics include:
- Nausea, malaise, and gastric upset.
- Prolonged use may affect the electrolyte balance in the body, causing nocturnal leg cramps.
- Blood calcium levels may be reduced – the importance of this in bone health has not been established.
- Gout in susceptible people.
- Blood cholesterol levels may rise.
- Allergic reactions have been reported – skin rashes, fever, interstitial nephritis.
- Occasionally the ability of the bone marrow to produce healthy blood cells has been affected.

C. Unwanted effects of progesterone are covered in detail on page 159.

D. Unwanted effects of the combined oral contraceptive include:
- Weight changes, most often weight gain.
- Benign and malignant liver tumours.
- It is now widely believed that users of the combined oral contraceptive experience blood clots more frequently than non-users. This makes risk of stroke and heart attack higher.

- Arterial thrombosis is also more common.

- Skin pigmentation may occur which may not resolve on stopping the treatment.

- Some chronic diseases may deteriorate such as: Depression; High blood pressure; Varicose veins; Otosclerosis; Diabetes mellitus; Multiple sclerosis; Migraine; Porphyria; Tetany; Disturbed liver function; Renal diseases; Uterine fibroids; Cardiovascular disease; Epilepsy; Gallstones; Asthma; Dry eyes.

- Numerous studies have been made on cancer risk. These appear to show that although taking the combined oral contraceptive may increase the risk of breast cancer, it offers protection against ovarian, colonic and endometrial cancers.

E. The use of HRT therapy has been discussed on page 160.

F. Gonadotrophin release hormone analogues may give the following unwanted effects:

- Because of the effect in lowering the level of female hormones, an imbalance occurs and male hormones predominate resulting in symptoms of masculinisation, such as hair growth, enlarged clitoris, etc.

- Induce a 'medical menopause' with potential unwanted effects as mentioned already on page 154.

- Must be given with progesterone and as women with PMS are susceptible to progesterone their symptoms will simply reappear.

G. Unwanted effects of antidepressants have been covered in detail on page 42.

H. Unwanted effects of anxiolytics are covered on page 18.

Non-drug ways to ease pre-menstrual syndrome

Certain foods have a profound effect on the natural balance of hormones. Many women have seen an improvement in their PMS symptoms, or even a complete disappearance of them, by introducing some dietary changes.

General dietary changes

Red meats, alcohol, nicotine, sugar, white flour and pasta products aggravate hormonal imbalance, so eat less or cut them out of your diet.

A diet low in animal fats and rich in green leafy vegetables and whole-grains improves hormone balance. If possible increase your intake of vegetables while making sure that your diet is low (<5%) in saturated fats.

Carbohydrates

Many women crave carbohydrates before a period. This has been found to raise the levels of natural mood enhancing hormones and therefore improve symptoms. Wholegrain cereals such as wholemeal bread, brown rice, wholemeal or vegetable pasta, wholegrain breakfast cereals such as Weetabix, oats, etc, appear to have the best effect. If you do not already include these in your diet, you may want to add some at each meal.

Oestrogenic foods

Include foods containing natural plant oestrogens in your diet. These have a beneficial effect on the body and have been found to reduce PMS. Quite how they work no one is yet sure – it may be that they reduce the effect of the oestrogens made in the body.

Foods containing natural plant oestrogens include:

- Peanuts
- Soya beans
- Tofu
- Black beans
- Lima beans

Calcium

It has been found that low levels of calcium intake made women more liable to mood swings, irritability, anxiety, headaches, backache, crying and depression. Their work performance and efficiency and memory were also reduced before menstruation. Try to make sure that you have at least one helping of foods high in calcium every day. These include:

- Sesame seeds
- Fish
- Dark green leafy vegetables
- Dried figs
- Tofu
- Legumes, such as baked beans, chickpeas, soya beans, etc

Manganese

If you skimp on foods containing manganese you could adversely affect your hormone levels. This may make your menstrual flow heavier than usual. Foods high in manganese include:

- Tea
- Fruits (especially pineapple)
- Vegetables
- Wholegrains
- Nuts and seeds

Vitamin B6

This is one of the few dietary components to be studied in depth, especially with regard to PMS. Nine randomised-controlled trials were considered with a total of 940 patients. Although many of the trials were not considered to be very good the authors concluded that 100mg of vitamin B6 significantly improved the symptoms of pre-menstrual syndrome in the vast majority of women.

Unwanted effects are uncommon but include headaches, nausea and upper and lower abdominal discomfort. This vitamin is found naturally in:

- Brewer's yeast
- Wheat bran
- Wholewheat products
- Liver and kidney
- Soya beans
- Cantaloupe melon
- Eggs

There has been some controversy about its safety. A report in 1980 suggested a link between high doses of vitamin B6 and damage to the nerves of the hands and feet leading to numbness and difficulty walking.

In 1997 the government restricted over-the-counter sales to doses of 50mg only. Unfortunately, women who suffer from PMS are unlikely to benefit from this dosage and probably need 100mg to show any improvement. The higher the dose taken the more likely unwanted effects are to occur. The most sensible way to judge if vitamin B6 will help you is to take it for six weeks and see if improvement occurs, then try to maintain levels by adding more B6-containing foods to your diet regularly.

Vitamin E

Several studies have found that vitamin E, 200-600mg per day, taken over several months may help symptoms of breast disease.

Oily Fish

A regular intake of oily fish or a supplement of fish oil, improves hormone balance as well as having a generalised anti-inflammatory action. Try to eat oily fish such as mackerel, salmon, herring, and tuna two to five times weekly or take a daily supplement of one (1000mg) fish oil capsule daily.

It is fashionable at the moment to eat a low fat diet but everyone needs some fat in order to produce the correct balance of hormones, maintain a normal menstrual cycle, ensure fertility and build healthy bones. The female hormone oestrogen is made in the body from fat and cholesterol. If you consume insufficient of the correct types of fat your body reduces oestrogen levels and this upsets the hormone balance. The best sorts of fats to eat are essential fatty acids such as olive oil, linseed oil, and oil of evening primrose. Hard fats, trans-fatty acids and hydrogenated fats as found in margarines are better avoided.

Oil of Evening Primrose

For centuries the essential fatty acid, oil of evening primrose, has been used to treat PMS. In some countries, such as the USA, the seeds are chewed. Luckily, it is possible to obtain this in capsule form in the UK. I recommend one 1000mg capsule daily, increasing to four capsules daily if the symptoms are felt to be developing. The oil is not advised for people with temporal lobe epilepsy and it interacts with anti-convulsant medication.

Salt
If you add a lot of salt to your cooking or add salt to your meals, try cutting this out. Excess salt can contribute to fluid retention making symptoms like bloating, irritability and breast pain worse. Processed food and cook-chill ready meals are invariably high in salt and should also be avoided.

Caffeine
Drinking four to eight cups of caffeine-containing drinks a day increases your chances of developing PMS tenfold! These include tea, coffee, cola drinks and chocolate. Carbonated drinks are, on the whole worse, as the caffeine is absorbed more rapidly from these. Women who experience PMS and fibrocystic breast disease seem to be much more sensitive to caffeine than other women. Try giving these drinks up for a few months to see if the symptoms diminish or vanish. Caffeine may also be found in some herbal tonics and over-the-counter drugs.

Exercise
Research shows that exercise decreases certain symptoms like breast tenderness and anxiety. Make an effort to do some regular exercise even if this is just getting out for a walk every day.

Psychology
Three out of five randomised controlled studies using psychological approaches to PMS management have demonstrated benefits.
If your symptoms continue or are very troublesome these herbal alternatives to conventional treatments are effective and safe.

Chasteberry/Monk's Pepper ~ *Vitex agnus castus*

Vitex agnus castus is actually the ripe fruit of a shrub from the Mediterranean regions. Its benefits come from its ability to influence the production of female hormones. Exhaustive research using biochemical and chemical techniques failed to reveal any hormonal component of Vitex at all. Researchers were convinced that the plant's natural chemicals were producing an effect on the body, possibly as a precursor to the hormones. In other words, Vitex encourages the body's glandular system to produce its own hormones.

It is not really known how Vitex works, but it is widely thought that it controls levels of progesterone and oestrogen by its effect on the anterior pituitary gland. Its presence regulates the two hormones produced there: follicle stimulating hormone (FSH) and luteinising hormone (LH). This enables the body to produce normal levels of the hormones progesterone and oestrogen, thereby relieving PMS symptoms.

The ability of Vitex to decrease excessive prolactin levels may benefit infertile women. Studies have shown that taking the herb once every morning over a period of several months encourages normal hormone levels and eases symptoms.

In a randomised controlled trial involving 170 women over three menstrual cycles this herb was found to be significantly more effective than placebo and few unwanted effects were reported.

In another trial a team of German doctors showed that *Vitex agnus castus* is superior to vitamin B6 in treating PMS. They conducted a double blind controlled trial involving 175 women over three menstrual cycles and concluded that, compared with vitamin B6, Vitex showed 'considerably more marked alleviation of typical PMS complaints'. Overall 77.1 per cent of the Vitex group reported improvement compared with 60.6 per cent of the vitamin B6 group.

I have used this herb for many years and find in many cases if it is used over a period of six cycles or so significant improvement occurs. Even if treatment ceases this often continues for six to 12 months or even longer.

Uses
- PMS
- Menopausal symptoms

Unwanted effects
- Skin rashes
- Headache
- Abdominal cramps
- Diarrhoea

Interactions with other herbs
- None

Interactions with other drugs
- Dopamine receptor antagonists

Contraindications
- Pregnancy, although it has been used to prevent miscarriage due to progesterone insufficiency in the first trimester
- Breastfeeding

Recommended dosage

Infusion	5 to 10g each morning
Tablets/capsules	200 to 400mg tab each morning
Tincture	5ml each morning in a glass of water

Ginkgo Biloba ~ *Ginkgo biloba*

This herb, which comprises the leaves of the maidenhair tree, is widely used especially on the continent for diminishing memory and concentation resulting from poor cerebral circulation and problems with the peripheral circulation such as intermittent claudication. Though not traditionally associated with the treatment of PMS a French study found ginkgo to be effective for congestive symptoms of PMS such as breast tenderness, ankle swelling and anxiety. Patients with more severe symptoms showed a clear statistical improvement.

Uses
- Congestive symptoms of PMS

Unwanted effects
- Abdominal discomfort has sometimes been reported

Interactions with other herbs
- None

Interactions with other drugs
- Warfarin and other anti-coagulants
- Aspirin
- Papaverine

Contraindications
- Epilepsy

Recommended dosage
Tablets – 3 x 120-240mg standardized extract of Ginkgo biloba daily
Or Tablets/capsules – 3 x 200-250mg Gingko leaf daily

Chinese Angelica ~ *Angelica sinensis*

In traditional Chinese medicine this is used to promote natural hormone balance. It is particularly useful where abdominal pain is experienced – see page 181.

Uses
- PMS

St John's Wort ~ *Hypericum perforatum*

This can be a useful addition to treatment for PMS where its anti-depressant action can play a role in reducing symptoms – see page 47.

Uses
- PMS

Motherwort ~ *Leonurus cardiaca*

This can help people who suffer from symptoms of anxiety during the pre-menstrual phase – see page 31.

Uses
- Anxiety

Lady's Mantle ~ *Alchemilla vulgaris*

The leaves are used medicinally. The generic name of this herb is derived from the Arabic word, Alkemelych (alchemy) in reference to the herb's exceptional healing qualities. It has a special affinity for women and is reported to be of benefit in treating PMS, dysmenorrhoea and menorrhagia (heavy periods). In clinical trials it inhibited breast tumour growth in mice and the animals' life expectancy was increased.

I can find much anecdotal evidence about this herb but no clinical trials have ever been carried out.

Uses
- PMS
- Heavy and painful periods

Unwanted effects
- None

Interactions with other herbs
- None

Interactions with other drugs
- None

Contraindications
- None

Recommended dosage
Dried herb – 2-4g as an infusion

15 | Vaginitis

He preferred to know the power of herbs and their value for curing purposes, and,
heedless of glory, to exercise that quiet art.   ~ Virgil, *Aeneid* (70-19BC)

Normally the vagina contains good bacteria (Döderlein's bacilli), which maintain a normal balance in the vagina and so keep infections at bay. These bacteria normally convert glucose into lactic acid so keeping the vagina at a slightly acidic pH. These healthy bacteria can be reduced by many factors – the most common are:

- Antibiotics
- Hormonal changes brought about by: Oral contraceptive pill; HRT; Menopause; Pregnancy.
- Diabetes mellitus
- Douching and using vaginal deodorants

When the levels of normal, healthy bacteria drop, unhealthy bacteria and yeasts can proliferate leading to vaginal discomfort and itching, or bacterial vaginosis and thrush (*Candida albicans*).

A. Clotrimazole is often used to treat thrush. It is convenient because only one pessary or application of cream needs to be inserted into the vagina to complete the treatment. It can be purchased from your local pharmacy.

B. Nystatin is another anti-fungal treatment available by prescription.

C. Diflucan is a tablet that treats thrush. It is only available on prescription. It should not be taken at the same time as the antihistamine Terfenadine.

Unwanted effects
A. Clotrimazole can cause the following:
- Localised burning and irritation

- It should not be used if the patient has: had more than two thrush infections in the last six months; a previous history of sexually transmitted disease; abnormal vaginal bleeding; fever or chills; nausea or vomiting; diarrhoea.

B. Nystatin can have the following unwanted effects:

- Localised irritation

C. Diflucan can have the following unwanted effects:

- Nausea, abdominal discomfort, diarrhoea and flatulence
- Headache
- Alopecia
- Disorders of the blood such as low platelet count
- Anaphylactic reactions
- Liver damage
- Skin rash (<1%) occasionally exfoliative dermatitis
- Special attention should be taken if it is administered with: Phenytoin; Oral contraceptives; Rifampicin; Terfenadine; Theophylline; Zidovudine; Tacrolimus; Hydrochlorothiazide; Sulphonylureas; Rifabutin; Anti-coagulants.

You can help to prevent thrush by:

Wearing loose clothes
Wear loose cotton clothes, avoid tights and other tight-fitting garments especially those made of synthetic fibres.

Bathing
Use your bidet to bathe yourself with saline. Dissolve half a cup of salt in a bidet full of warm water and immerse the vagina and vulva in it. Insert your fingers into the vagina to allow the warm salt water in, then remove your fingers and relax in the water for 10-15 minutes.

Drying
When you have finished bathing or showering you may be too sore to dry yourself thoroughly. This is unfortunate as the unfriendly bacteria and

yeasts need moisture to survive – this creates the environment for their optimum growth. Give yourself a blow dry with a hairdryer! Take care though – it must not be set too hot, and electrical appliances should never be used where there is water because of the risk of electrocution.

Yoghurt

Eat a cupful of live organic yoghurt daily. If you can't take dairy products, soya, sheeps' milk and goats' milk products are widely available. Acidophilus tablets are available as an alternative.

Allergy

Some people are very sensitive to contact with soaps, bubble bath, perfumed or unperfumed talc or even coloured toilet paper, dyed underwear, condoms and lubricants. Be suspicious if your problem is recurrent – you should be able to determine what is causing the irritation by a process of trial and error.

Essential oils

You may prefer to bathe using essential oils rather than bubble bath. Some are known to be fungicidal. These include German chamomile, cinnamon leaf, tagetes and pine.

Diabetes

Ask your GP to check that you have not developed diabetes. A finger-prick test will establish your level of blood sugar. Some GPs prefer to do a urine test or you may be referred to a hospital pathology laboratory for a glucose tolerance test.

Vitamin C

Take 500 mg vitamin C twice daily. As well as improving your immunity, it will increase the acidity of the vagina and suppress growth of unwanted bacteria.

Zinc

Take a zinc supplement – it plays an important role in your immune system. Taking zinc lozenges for a month may increase your immunity to candida and other unwanted bacteria

These alternative treatments have been shown to alleviate thrush:

Lavender ~ *Lavendula officinalis*

Lavender has a gentle antibacterial and anti-fungal action and is very effective in treating thrush. It is also mildly sedative and reduces anxiety. Lavender is readily available as an essential oil. It is dealt with in detail on page 35.

Lavender has a low toxicity but significant antibacterial action.

Uses
- Vaginitis

Unwanted effects
- None

Contraindications
- Pregnancy

Interactions with other herbs/drugs/vitamins
- None

Recommended dosage
Pessaries made with 25g of cocoa butter and 10 drops of essential oil of lavender – Insert one each night for six nights.

Tea Tree ~ *Melaleuca alternifolia*

Tea tree is the essential oil distilled from the leaves of the tree, *Melaleuca alternifolia*. It has significant antibacterial, antiviral and antifungal properties. Native Australians have used it for centuries and now a large amount of research, which confirms its effectiveness, has been carried out in Australian Universities. Tea tree has already been mentioned on page 150.

Uses
- Bacterial vaginosis
- Thrush

Unwanted effects
- Localised discomfort/burning

Contraindications
- Pregnancy and breastfeeding
- Allergy to this herb

Interactions with other herbs/drugs/vitamins
- None

Recommended dosage
A tampon soaked in a 40 percent solution of tea tree oil and inserted for 24 hrs once a week for six weeks.

Or wash with a 1 percent solution (that is 5ml, or 1 teaspoonful, in 500ml water) twice daily.

Or insert a pessary made with 25g cocoa butter and 10 drops of tea tree oil each night for six nights.

Witch Hazel ~ *Hamamelis virginiana*

Witch hazel is obtained from a tree native to North Eastern United States and Canada. It is now widely found in European gardens. It is very astringent and also bacteriostatic. In cases of vaginal infection it can be very beneficial in reducing infection as well as relieving tissue swelling which causes an aching and dragging sensation. Witch hazel has been further discussed on page 146.

Witch hazel contains two or three volatile oils and also has a high tannin content, this gives it its astringency, which also aids its healing.

Medicinal uses
- Bacterial vaginosis

Unwanted effects

- None

Contraindications

- None

Interactions with other herbs/drugs/vitamins

- None

Recommended dosage

Insert a pessary made from 55g of cocoa butter and 10g of finely ground bark of witch hazel. Repeat every night for six nights.

16 | Benign Prostatic Hypertrophy (BHP)

First the word, then the plant, lastly the knife.

~ Aesculapius of Thassaly c1200BC

Prostate problems are on the increase. If you are a man aged between 40 and 60 you have a 40-60 per cent chance of having benign enlargement of the prostate gland. The older you become, the greater the chance of developing a problem. As our population ages there are potentially more men with prostate disorders.

As its name suggests BPH is a non-malignant condition but the symptoms caused by it can be very troublesome and affect the sufferer's quality of life.

The prostate gland is a small gland, normally about the size of a horse chestnut, encircling the urethra (the tube through which the urine is passed out of the body). It produces most of the fluid in semen and therefore in the ejaculate. It comprises two lateral and a median (middle) lobe.

It is thought that the production of lower levels of the male hormone, testosterone, with increasing age and/or increasing weight leads to production of dihydrotestosterone. This in turn stimulates the prostate gland leading to over-production of prostate cells and a slowly enlarging gland. Being overweight and having excess fatty tissue also alters the body's hormone profile.

The degree of enlargement is variable but it is usually between 60-100g and seldom more than 200g, usually involving the lateral and median lobes. The gland remains firm and rubbery but there are may be cystic areas and places where the prostatic tissue dies (infarction) and secondary infection can also occur.

Caucasians are more likely to be affected than Asians or Negroes. The reason for this is not known but dietary habits may be relevant.

Men who are overweight, with a 43inch or larger waist, are 50 per cent more likely to experience prostate enlargement and to require surgery for this complaint. Unfortunately, obesity also leads to more post-operative complications.

Considering the prevalence of BPH, it seems likely that almost every man will develop a prostate disorder sooner or later – the majority of these will seek treatment from their family doctor or an urologist. It is estimated that while drugs help 60 per cent of men with this problem, plant-based medicines like saw palmetto may help as many as 90 per cent.

It is important to exclude malignant disease of the prostate when symptoms are present so patients should not attempt to make the diagnosis themselves but seek a professional opinion.

Typical symptoms of an enlarged prostate gland include:

- Passing urine more frequently than normal. Normally urine is passed approximately every three hours; in BPH it may be more frequently than two hourly.

- The sudden uncontrollable desire to urinate.

- A weak or intermittent stream of urine.

- You might have to strain to pass urine.

- An inability to voluntarily arrest your urinary stream.

- A sense that you have incompletely emptied your bladder.

- Dribbling when you have finished passing urine.

- Loss of libido or impotence.

- Urinary infections are more common.

- Getting up in the night to pass water is characteristic.

- An inability to hold your urine, ie incontinence, may occur.

- Occasionally blood occurs in the urine due to rupture of a vein in the enlarged prostate tissue or possibly because of infection in the urine.

- Rarely the complete inability to pass urine occurs. The use of some stronger painkillers such as dihydrocodeine may precipitate this.

Sometimes complications occur as long-term consequences of this condition.

- Prostatitis – a painful inflammation of the prostate gland.
- Bladder stones.
- Chronic renal failure – usually to suffer this you will have had BPH for a long time and it will have caused back pressure on the kidneys.

Drugs used in the treatment of BPH:

A. α-Blockers (Terazosin; Doxasocin; Alfuzosin; Tamsulosin) – these are more effective in reducing symptoms than 5α reductase inhibitors. They work by relaxing the muscle in the urethra, thus improving urinary flow. They do nothing to correct the hormonal dysfunction that leads to this problem.

B. 5α reductase inhibitors (Finasteride) – this drug is a competitive inhibitor of the enzyme that metabolises testosterone into dihydroxy-testosterone. Patients need to take it continually for six to 12 months before they see any improvement in their symptoms. Prostatic size may reduce by 20 per cent; corresponding urine flow was shown to increase by up to 17 per cent.

A. α-Blockers are known to have the following unwanted effects:

- Dizziness, light-headedness and fainting
- Low blood pressure brought on by a change of posture from sitting or lying down to standing
- Palpitations
- Breathlessness
- Blurred vision
- Weight gain and tissue swelling
- Weakness/muscle pains
- Vertigo
- Pain in the extremities
- Persistent running nose/sinusitis/nosebleeds
- Sexual difficulties including abnormal ejaculation and decreased libido

- Depression and nervousness
- There have been at least two cases of severe allergic reaction following administration of this drug

Less common side effects associated with this drug include:
- Constipation or diarrhoea
- Dyspepsia, flatulence, vomiting
- Arthritis, gout
- Tinnitus
- Increased cough
- Urinary frequency and incontinence
- Abnormal heart rhythms
- Neck and shoulder pains
- Fever and flu-like symptoms
- Insomnia

B. 5α reductase inhibitors are known to have the following unwanted effects:
- Decreased libido
- Impotence
- Decreased volume of ejaculate
- Breast enlargement or tenderness
- Possible birth defects, if sexual intercourse results in a partner's pregnancy

Lifestyle changes which can help:

Weight

Lose weight if you need to – this will improve symptoms in several ways. Achieving a normal weight takes pressure off the bladder and helps to alter the hormone changes that lead to enlargement of the gland.

Fluid

When urinary problems occur there is a tendency to cut down on fluid intake. If anything you should increase the amount that you drink. Remember to drink more in hot weather and before and after exercise.

Water is undoubtedly the best fluid to drink. Alcoholic drinks and caffeine-containing beverages can result in a sudden increase in urinary output and may occasionally result in a sudden inability to pass urine (acute retention of urine). Aim for a minimum of two litres of fluid evenly spaced throughout the day. Drinking a glass of cranberry juice daily has been shown to decrease your risk of developing a urinary infection.

Diet

Some foods appear to have a beneficial effect on the prostate gland. These include tomatoes, nuts (especially hazelnuts and pecans), wholewheat products and fruits such as kiwi fruit, mango and papaya.

Tomatoes are especially beneficial for the prostate gland as they contain the natural chemical, lycopene. Studies of diet show that men who eat tomatoes regularly, (three to four tomato products a week) have a lower incidence of prostate problems. It is now possible to buy a supplement with a high lycopene content. Lycopene is also found in watermelon.

Research has shown that beta-sitosterol taken three times a day reduced the size of the prostate gland. This can be found in various foods such as garlic, beetroot, oats, soya products, peas, peanuts and other legumes, olives, cherries, buckwheat, corn and chocolate. It is also present in many herbs such as yarrow, St John's wort, dandelion, fenugreek, red clover, liquorice and hops.

Linseed

A supplement of linseed oil/flaxseed oil (2000mg daily) has been used to reduce symptoms in BPH. In 1941, 19 men were given this oil. Over several weeks they experienced reduction in night-time urination, less fatigue, increased libido, better stream and reduction in prostate size. No problems have been reported with regard to taking this supplement.

Quercetin

Foods high in quercetin appear to help some prostate disorders. Quercetin is found in a large variety of foods including onions, apples, kale and tea. Thirty-nine men with long-standing prostate problems took 500mg of quercetin twice daily for two weeks. Sixty per cent saw an improvement in symptoms.

Zinc

Eat foods high in zinc – these include shellfish (especially oysters), meat, liver, wheat germ, eggs and ground mustard. Zinc is essential to maintain enzyme systems and a healthy immune response within the body. There is much evidence to confirm that efficient production of sex hormones in normal amounts can only occur in the presence of adequate zinc levels. To function correctly the prostate gland needs to use ten times more than any other organ in the body. Processing foods depletes it of this mineral. Levels are low in foods grown in nutrient poor soil anyway and it is likely that deficiencies will occur. It has been estimated that 90 per cent of the population of industrialised nations eat a diet deficient in zinc. If you wish to take a supplement <15mg is recommended in a multi-mineral tablet to prevent imbalances. It should include:

- Zinc
- Copper
- Calcium
- Magnesium
- Phosphorus
- Vitamin A

Green tea

Recent animal studies suggest that drinking green tea may help to reduce the size of the prostate gland and possibly prevent prostate cancer.

Pumpkin seeds

Eat a handful of pumpkin seeds (*Cucurbita pepo*) every day. These are the traditional treatment for BPH in Eastern Europe where men were recommended to eat a handful of seeds per day throughout adulthood. Pumpkin seeds work in a variety of ways:

- Pumpkin seed oil is a natural diuretic.
- Pumpkin seeds contain curcurbitacins – these phyto-chemicals reduce the size of the prostate by preventing transformation of testosterone into dihydrotestosterone.
- Their high zinc content aids in reducing the size of the prostate gland.

- Pumpkin seeds are high in the amino acids alanine, glycine and glutamic acid. High doses of these amino acids have been shown to reduce the size of the prostate gland.

Rye grass pollen extract
Try taking this supplement – it decreases the need to urinate at night and improves general symptoms without significant unwanted effects.

Fibre
Adopt a high fibre diet – keeping your bowels open is a way of avoiding problems with fully emptying the bladder.

Diabetes mellitus
Prostate problems appear to be more prevalent in men with maturity onset diabetes mellitus, because excess insulin levels can also stimulate growth of prostatic tissue. Keeping your blood sugar levels under control is therefore of paramount importance. Ask your GP or practice nurse for advice.

Surgery
Another available option is surgery. It may be helpful in the short term and is certainly indispensable in the treatment of acute urinary retention. It does, of course, do nothing to correct underlying biochemical abnormalities and symptoms can recur. Ten per cent of patients require a repeat operation within 10 years.

Trans urethral resection of the prostate (TURP) was developed in the USA in the 1920s. It is a commonly used surgical technique that involves passing a tube, called a resectoscope, into the bladder through the penile urethra while the patient is under general or local anaesthetic. This enables the surgeon to scrape away excess tissue and alleviate the obstruction responsible for most of the symptoms.

TURP relieves symptoms in 70-95 per cent of patients depending on the expertise of the surgeon. Mortality rate is between one and 10 per cent depending on the hospital.

Early complications are:

- Failure to pass urine
- Bleeding (in 5 to15 per cent of patients)
- Retention of blood clots in the bladder

More long-term side effects are not unusual:

- Approximately 5 per cent of patients suffer from stricture formation – scarring in the urethra that eventually leads to an inability to pass urine so this area must be dilated regularly.

- 15 per cent of patients suffer from erectile dysfunction (impotence).

- 5 per cent have urinary incontinence.

- 70 per cent suffer from retrograde ejaculation (dry ejaculation).

It is, of course, possible to have more than one side effect at a time.

Surprisingly, although doctors thought that early surgical intervention in BPH would help patients to live longer and maintain their good health, research done by Dr J E Wennberg at Dartmouth Medical School USA in 1990 showed that pre-emptive surgery actually lowered life expectancy. He determined that patients who had undergone TURP were more likely to suffer a heart attack than those who chose an alternative method of treatment.

Prostatectomy – or removal of the prostate gland through an incision in the lower abdomen – is usually reserved for patients with very large prostate glands. It has a significantly higher mortality rate.

Transurethral microwave thermotherapy (TUMT) uses heat to destroy excess tissue. At the moment it is largely an experimental technique, although it has been found to significantly reduce symptoms.

Dilatation of the urethra using a balloon at high pressure. This has been used in patients with smaller prostate glands.

Various types of laser therapy. This appears to be effective and safe but more research is underway.

Urethral stents are small tubes inserted into the urethra, usually on a permanent basis, to relieve obstruction. This tends to be reserved for those who are too ill for other procedures and cannot wait for medical treatments to take effect.

If your symptoms continue or are very troublesome there are a number of herbal alternatives to conventional treatments that are effective and safe.

Saw Palmetto ~ *Serenoa serrulata/repens*

This is a small palm tree that grows in south eastern USA particularly around Florida and the Everglades. Seminole Indians ate saw palmetto seed as a food and later realised its medicinal potential. There is considerable evidence that this herb is effective in treating BPH. It is also called Sabal.

Saw palmetto works because it contains a compound that inhibits the action of the enzyme testosterone – 5-alpha-reductase that turns testosterone into Dihydrotestosterone (DHT). Saw palmetto also blocks DHT from binding in the prostate. Because of the nature of the problem, treatment will need to be taken indefinitely.

It is preferable to have lower levels of this hormone as it prevents over-stimulation and consequent enlargement of the gland and may help to reduce the risk of prostate cancer. As yet there is no research into this but epidemiological studies show a lower incidence of prostate cancer in countries where men have naturally lower levels of this hormone.

A clinical trial found that patients' improvement when taking saw palmetto was better than in men taking placebo. A further international study of over 1000 men compared saw palmetto with finasteride. Both drug and the herb relieved symptoms in over 60 per cent of men, but saw palmetto worked faster and patients had less problems of impotence and loss of libido.

A placebo controlled study conducted in Chicago, USA, involving 85 men over six months showed significant improvement in urinary symptoms in the group taking saw palmetto.

In 1984 a double-blind study showed that saw palmetto had a dramatic effect on urine flow for men with BPH. It also proved more effective than finasteride in treating symptoms. In a study of 305 patients with mild to moderate BPH, patients were given 160mg of saw palmetto twice daily for three months. There was an 88 per cent success rate.

Further trials compared saw palmetto and found similar improvement with both products but significantly fewer side effects in men taking the herbal preparation.

A clinical trial involving 2000 Germans with BPH produced substantial easing of their symptoms.

Uses
- BPH

Unwanted effects
- These are low (1.8 per cent v 11 per cent with finasteride and v 10 per cent with terazosin)
- Gastro-intestinal disturbance – this resolves if the medication is taken with meals

Interactions with other herbs
- None

Interactions with other drugs
- Alpha adrenergic blockers
- Androgens (male hormones)

Contraindications
- None

Recommended dosage
Capsules/tablets of saw palmetto – 320mg standardised extract daily

Stinging Nettle Root ~ *Urtica dioica radix*

Usually the aerial parts of the nettle are used, but for prostate disease an extract of stinging nettle roots has been successful in treating BPH. It is known to contain beta-sitosterol.

Researchers gave men with BPH two to three teaspoonfuls of nettle root extract – it significantly reduced their need to get up in the night to pass urine and increased the volume and maximum flow of urine in men with early stage BPH.

One trial compared saw palmetto and Urtica extract with finasteride in BPH. The trial recruited 543 patients to measure maximum urinary flow after 24 weeks therapy. Volume of urine and time taken to empty the bladder were also taken into account as well as quality of life. The clinical results were the same in both groups; the most notable difference was the lower incidence of adverse effects with the plant-based medicine group particularly in the areas of diminished ejaculation volume, impotence and headache.

In a double blind placebo-controlled clinical trial of extract of nettle root in Germany, hesitancy and post micturition dribbling improved by 83 per cent. Maximum urine flow was increased by 87 per cent. Overall urinary problems were reduced in 91 per cent of patients.

Uses
- BPH
- Irritable bladder

Unwanted effects
- Contact with fresh nettles can cause a rash
- Occasional mild gastro-intestinal complaints

Interactions with other herbs
- None

Interactions with other drugs
- None

Contraindications
- None

Recommended dosage
Root extract   2-3 teaspoons or 120mg nettle root extract daily
Tincture   2-4ml three times daily

Liquorice ~ *Glycyrrhiza glabra*

Liquorice contains a compound that prevents conversion of testosterone into dihydroxytestosterone. It also contains significant amounts of β-sitosterol which reduces the size of the prostate gland. Care is needed in its use and the type of patient for whom it is advised. Liquorice is discussed in more detail on page 101.

Red Stinkwood ~ *Prunus africana*

This plant, formerly known as *Pygeum africanum*, is indigenous to southern Africa where it grows at high altitudes. It contains beta sitosterol and possibly terpenoids which contribute to its beneficial effect on the prostate gland. This includes reducing the size of the gland, lowering cholesterol levels within the prostate (this reduces male hormone production) and levels of prolactin (this also reduces the level of male hormones within the prostate), and reducing inflammation.

In three double blind, placebo-controlled trials, men who used this herb showed a marked improvement in symptoms and reduction in prostate size.

In 1997 some 3200 to 4900 tonnes of bark were exported for medicinal use mainly for the treatment of BPH.

Unfortunately through high demand for medicinal use it is now an endangered species. I do not prescribe this plant and strongly suggest that others refrain from using it until cultivated sources become available.

17 | Urinary tract infections

Venienti occurrite morbo (Meet the disease as it approaches)

~ Persius (34-62AD)

Urinary tract infections are the most commonly seen in general practice and can result in a large number of hospital admissions as well as a significant reduction in quality of life.

Symptoms of urinary tract infection (UTI) include:

- Pain on passing urine
- Passing urine more frequently than usual
- Rising in the night to pass urine
- Lower abdominal pain

There may also be

- Blood in the urine
- Fever
- Back pain

Fifty per cent of women experience a urinary tract infection, most commonly cystitis, at some time in their lives. Of these 50 per cent or half – that is a quarter of all women, have frequent or recurrent urinary infections. In addition, in women, hormonal changes can relax smooth muscle in the urethra or make the terminal third of the urethra less resistant to infection.

In men cystitis is less common due to anatomical differences, most notably the longer urethra that prevents bacteria ascending to the bladder so easily.

There are times when bladder infections are more common in both men and women:

CANCER: HERBS IN HOLISTIC HEALTHCARE

- At the onset of sexual activity, known as 'honeymoon cystitis' in women.

- When insufficient fluids are taken either due to nausea and vomiting or loss of appetite.

- If diarrhoea is present.

- When sufficient fluids are taken but losses have increased – for instance in cases of fever or in a hot climate (or even a hot ward or room).

- When there is an enlarged prostate gland (see chapter 16).

- Self catheterisation or catheterisation by a health professional.

Most patients who see their GP or hospital doctor with cystitis will be treated with antibiotics immediately. However some people experience unpleasant adverse effects:

- Gastrointestinal tract disturbance – minor changes, such as nausea, vomiting, diarrhoea, abdominal pain and difficulty swallowing are common. Patients prescribed more than two courses of antibiotic over a three to five year period are 60 per cent more likely to develop Crohn's disease. Occasionally more serious adverse reactions affecting the gut have been reported (pseudomembranous colitis and haemorrhagic colitis).

- Skin rashes, itching, and nettle rash. Occasional severe reactions and dermatitis can occur. Sensitivity to sunlight is not uncommon. Note that skin reactions may not manifest themselves for up to six months after taking antibiotics.

- Changes to the eye – these are very rare, but can be serious and result in blindness.

- Chest pains, cardiac arrhythmias and palpitations have been seen in patients taking some antibiotics, most notably erythromycin. Enlargement of the heart may be associated with the use of some antibiotics.

- Vaginal thrush – at its mildest a slight discharge and some irritation, but it can result in a severe burning feeling and a thick unpleasant irritant discharge (see page 199).

- Oral thrush can lead to a sore mouth and difficulty swallowing – it can be hard to eradicate especially in debilitated patients.
- Occasionally patients develop a black hairy tongue after antibiotic treatment.
- Acute allergic reactions that may show themselves as swelling and acute breathlessness.
- Kidney damage has been reported very occasionally.
- Effects on the nervous system but these are uncommon. They include headache, visual disturbance, dizziness and convulsions.
- Jaundice and pancreatitis have been seen occasionally but are more likely if the patient has taken chemotherapeutic agents. Transient abnormalities of liver enzymes occur sometimes but are not thought to be significant.
- Changes in the blood have occurred, possibly due to the antibiotic interfering in the production of blood cells. These changes may include a low white cell count and/or low platelet count.
- Some antibiotics, such as trimethoprim, interfere with the absorption of folic acid. Others, for example tetracyclines and sulphonamides, interact with vitamin C. This is unlikely to cause major problems in the short term but if extended courses of these antibiotics or long-term therapy is considered this should be taken into consideration.
- Some antibiotics interfere with absorption of minerals into the body, most notably potassium, iron, zinc, calcium and magnesium.

If you are already debilitated by illness or chemotherapy/radiotherapy even a minor side effect can significantly lower quality of life and alter your outlook and psychological response to treatment.

Often, simple measures adopted early will forestall an attack:
Increase fluids
Drink, drink, drink! Unless there are medical reasons why you should not increase your fluid intake, drink one 200ml glass of fluid every half-hour during waking hours, up to a maximum of 2000ml daily. Avoid acidic drinks such as orange squash/juice or lemon barley drink. Filtered or mineral (non-carbonated) water is best. Alcohol, tea (unless very weak or herbal – not fruit), cola drinks and coffee should also be avoided.

Sweeteners
Avoid drinks, yoghurts and any other products containing aspartame and saccharin as these irritate the bladder. The combination of these two sweetening agents can 'scald' the inside of the bladder, making symptoms much worse.

Clothing
Wear clothes that don't restrict the genital area. Anything with a tight crotch can put pressure on the urethral opening and this can force bacteria back up into the bladder. Pure cotton underwear is better as it is absorptive, keeps the area dry and prevents the growth of bacteria.

Sex
There is a definite association of UTIs and sexual activity for some women. The usual missionary position can cause friction around the urethra making infection more likely. Contraceptive diaphragms with a hard rim also traumatise the urethra – it is usually possible to change these for a smaller one – say under 65mm. Using condoms has also been associated with an increase in the incidence of UTIs – if you are using a spermicidally treated condom try changing to a lubricated one and *vice versa*.

Tampons
If you regularly get an infection around period time, the problem may be your tampon. Super-size absorbent tampons can compress the bladder neck and alter urine flow so that you can't completely empty your bladder. The answer is to change your tampon before every visit to the lavatory to empty your bladder.

Green tea
The polyphenols in green tea have antibacterial action. Drink several cups per day, but bear in mind that it does contain caffeine, but not as much as coffee.

Alkalinise
Take half a teaspoonful of bicarbonate of soda in a little water, provided you have no kidney problems. This drink will 'alkalinize' your urine. Most bacteria that cause urinary infections prefer to grow in acid urine – their growth will slow appreciably in an alkaline environment, giving you the chance to flush them out.

Soak
If you have lower abdominal cramps sit in a warm bath to which you have added five drops of oil of lavender, black pepper, juniper berry, sandalwood, tea tree or niaouli.

Painkiller
Take a mild painkiller, such as white willow tablets, if you have lower abdominal pain – see page 84.

Warmth
Place a hot water bottle on your lower abdomen to help relax the muscles of the bladder and take away some of the spasm that makes you feel as if you want to pass water all the time.

In cases when a clinical and/or bacteriological diagnosis of cystitis has been made and measures outlined above have not brought relief there are several herbal medicines with powerful antibacterial action that work quickly and effectively against *E coli* and the other bacteria that commonly cause urinary tract infections. I would, however, suggest that a time limit is put on their use. In my practice I specify that if the patient is no better in 48 hours or develops other symptoms such as fever, abdominal or back pain, which suggests worsening of the illness or a kidney infection, then they begin an antibiotic straight away. In my experience very few patients need to change from their herbal prescription.

Cranberry ~
Vaccinium macrocarpon (V. oxycoccos) (V. erythrocarpum)

In North America, cranberry juice has been used to treat and prevent urinary tract infections for hundreds of years. If you have experienced cystitis in the past, then drink a glass of cranberry juice daily. This is believed to work by making the bladder surface more slippery so that bacteria can't cling to the lining so attacks are prevented. Blueberries are also effective.

A double blind, placebo controlled trial was conducted at Harvard Medical School in the USA. Researchers asked patients either to drink 300ml cranberry juice per day or 300ml placebo that looked like and tasted like the real juice over a six-month period. Those who had drunk cranberry juice were nearly half as likely to have developed a UTI or have been prescribed antibiotics for a UTI during this period.

A recent randomised trial in Oulu, Finland, confirmed cranberry's effectiveness. This time it was administered as a cranberry/lingonberry juice. Researchers found that patients who took the concentrate daily reduced their recurrences of urinary tract infection by about half compared to the control group who took a lactobacillus drink that had no effect on recurrences.

Uses
- Prevention of urinary tract infections

Unwanted effects
- None

Interactions with other herbs
- None

Interactions with other drugs
- None

Contraindications
- None

Recommended dosage

Tablets/capsules   2-3 x 400mg daily

Decoction   a handful of berries simmered for 30-45minutes, 3-4 cups daily

Fruit juice   200ml undiluted cranberry juice daily

Thyme ~ *Thymus vulgaris*

This well-known garden herb is widely used in the kitchen. Most households have dried thyme in their store cupboard – however the main effective agent is essential oil of thyme or thymol which is lost from the dried herb quite quickly in a warm kitchen.

Thymol is a powerful antibacterial with bactericidal properties, 40 times more potent than phenol, but so gentle that it can be safely put in the eyes. It has a special affinity for the respiratory and urinary tracts. If ingested as an infusion or tincture 50 per cent will be excreted in the breath, the other 50 per cent in the urine. It is particularly good if used as a preventative and makes an acceptable evening drink. It can be taken either sweetened or unsweetened using sugar or honey.

Uses
- Cystitis
- Bronchitis

Unwanted effects
- Systemic allergic effects have been reported leading to oedema and difficulty breathing

Interactions with other herbs
- None

Interactions with other drugs
- None

Contraindications
- Conditions where the gut is very sensitive such as IBS and inflammatory bowel disease.
- Pregnancy

Recommended dosage

Dried herb	1 to 3 teaspoons daily
Capsules	1.5mg daily
Fresh herb juice	30ml daily
Tincture BHP (1983) 1:5 in 45% alcohol	3 to 18ml daily
Liquid extract	30 to 180 drops daily

Buchu ~ *Barosma betulina*

The aerial parts of this plant are used medicinally. Buchu is well known as a safe urinary antiseptic and general tonic. It acts to eliminate mucus and reduce inflammation and has been used in South Africa for hundreds of years. It is now grown commercially and is available worldwide.

Uses

- Urinary infections
- Irritable bladder
- Prostatitis

Unwanted effects

- Diarrhoea and other gastro-intestinal disturbance
- Increased menstrual flow
- Raised liver enzymes

Interactions with other herbs

- None

Interactions with other drugs

- Warfarin and other anti-coagulants

Contraindications

- Pregnancy and breastfeeding
- Liver damage

Recommended dosage

Dried herb	3 teaspoons daily
Tincture BHC 1:5 in 60% alcohol	3 to 6ml daily
Liquid extract BHC 1:1 in 90% alcohol	1.5 to 4.5ml daily

Bearberry ~ *Arctostaphylos uva-ursi*

This is a trailing evergreen shrub of the heather family with shiny red berries. The leaves are used medicinally. Bearberry is known to have antibiotic effects and urine sterilising properties. It is also slightly diuretic.

Maximum antibacterial activity is expected three to four hours after administration in an alkaline urine. The tannins in the herb act as an astringent, coagulating the proteins on the bladder tissue and reducing inflammation. This helps to reduce feelings of urgency and pain.

Administration of this herb may turn the urine dark green!

Main uses

- Cystitis
- Vaginitis

Unwanted effects

- Gastro-intestinal symptoms such as nausea

Interactions with other herbs

- None

Interactions with other drugs

- Will be antagonised by any drug that acidifies the urine
- May increase the gastrointestinal irritation of NSAIs
- May antagonise the diuretic effects of thiazide and loop diuretics

Contraindications

- Pregnancy and breastfeeding
- Kidney disorders – theoretical
- Digestive disorders – theoretical
- Children under 12 years of age
- Conditions where the gut is very sensitive such as IBS and inflammatory bowel disease.

Recommended dosage

The urine must be alkaline for this herb to work effectively. Citrus fruits and drinks, pickles, vitamin C and meals containing large amounts of meat should be avoided.

Dried herb	1g daily
Liquid extract BHC 1:1 in 25% alcohol	4.5 to 7.5ml daily
Tincture BHC 1:5 in 25% alcohol	6 to 12ml daily

Golden Seal ~ *Hydrastis canadensis*

The rhizome of this plant is used medicinally. One of its other names is yellow root because it stains work surfaces and clothes yellow. The main constituents of this well-known herb are hydrastine and berberine, which give it its bright yellow colour. In many research programmes they have been shown to be anti-inflammatory and antibacterial as well as anti-haemorrhagic.

Hydrastis has an especial affinity for the mucus membranes. It has been suggested that as well as its antibacterial effect it acts on mucosal surfaces by coagulating proteins, reducing congestion secondary to inflammation. Golden seal has already been discussed in detail on page 108.

Uses

- Cystitis
- Vaginitis
- Digestive disturbance such as gastritis

226

Cornsilk ~ *Zea mais*

The delicate silky fronds of fresh corn-on-the-cob have been used for urinary problems for millennia. They are actually the stigmata and styles of the plant. When taken as a tea or tincture they have little flavour but exert a soothing effect on the lining of the bladder and urinary tubules, relieving irritation and frequency. This is better mixed with one of the urinary antibacterials such as golden seal or bearberry.

Uses
- Cystitis
- Urethritis
- Kidney stones

Unwanted effects
- None.

Interactions with other herbs
- None

Interactions with other drugs
- Warfarin and other anti-coagulants

Contraindications
- Diabetes mellitus (may lower blood sugar)

Recommended dosage

Dried herb	6 to 24g daily
Liquid extract	15 to 30ml daily
Tincture	15 to 45ml daily

Horsetail ~ *Equisetum arvensis*

Horsetail is a primitive plant, a descendant of the huge trees of the Palaeozoic era (600-375 million years ago). The high mineral content of its aerial parts makes it an excellent astringent or styptic herb for the urinary tract especially where cystitis or urethritis has caused severe inflammation and bleeding. It stops bleeding and helps to speed the repair of damaged connective tissue.

Horsetail has a high silica content (70 per cent) and also contains other essential minerals. Silica preserves the elasticity of connective tissue and controls absorption of calcium. It is an essential ingredient of bones, nails, hair and teeth and is therefore also useful where there is risk of osteoporosis.

Uses
- Cystitis
- Urethritis
- Prostatitis
- Osteoporosis

Unwanted effects
- None

Interactions with other herbs.
- *Digitalis purpurea* (Foxglove)

Interactions with other drugs
- Digoxin and other cardiac glycosides

Contraindications
- Heart disease

Recommended dosage

Dried herb	3 to 12g daily
Fresh herb juice	30ml daily
Liquid extract BHC 1:1 in 25% alcohol	3 to 12ml daily
Tincture 1:4 in 25% alcohol	6 to 15ml daily

Juniper ~ *Juniperis communis*

Juniper is usually taken as a tea made from the aerial parts of the tree – it has the distinctive smell and taste of gin! This well-known strong urinary antiseptic has been used in the USA for over 200 years. It is known to promote the flow of urine and increase the elimination of acid metabolites.

Uses
- Cystitis

Unwanted effects
- None

Interactions with other herbs
- None

Interactions with other drugs
- None

Contraindications
- Pregnancy
- Heavy menstrual periods
- Kidney infection/pyelonephritis
- Kidney disease, such as Bright's disease
- Conditions where the gut is very sensitive such as IBS and inflammatory bowel disease.

Recommended dosage
To be used for up to 14 days:

Dried herb	6 to 30g daily
Tincture BHP 1:5 in 45% alcohol	3 to 6ml daily

18 | Impotence

In human intimacy there is a secret boundary; neither the experience of being in love nor passion can cross it, though lips be joined together in awful silence, and the heart break asunder with love.
~ Anna Akhmatova 1899-1966

There can be few more distressing symptoms than impotence especially as this will involve your partner as well, and can put pressure on even the closest relationship. Failure to either achieve or maintain an erection can be a humiliating experience even if you have never had a sexual problem before, and even if there does not seem to be a good reason for your failure. We know that happiness in love helps to promote good health.

Impotence (erectile dysfunction) affects millions of men worldwide – possibly as many as 52 per cent of all men between 40 and 75.

There has been much hype about drugs to treat impotence over the past few years. One good effect is to bring the topic of male impotence into open discussion. Formerly men believed that impotence was something to be ashamed of and if they had a problem with potency they were less of a man. We now know that lack of libido is a common problem both in men and women at any age and as our population grows older it is likely to become more common.

Many drugs are anaphrodisiacs, that is, they decrease sexual potency. If you are taking any of these drugs do not stop them but discuss your sexual problems with your GP or oncologist who will probably be able to suggest a change in drug regime. These include:

- Antihistamines – see pages 59 and 114.
- Tranquillisers and hypnotics (sleeping pills) – see page18.
- Diuretics
- Proton pump inhibitors, taken to lower levels of stomach acid in cases of indigestion – see page 92.

- Statins, taken to lower cholesterol
- Domperidone taken for nausea – see page 114.
- β-blockers, used to treat high blood pressure – see page 22.
- Antidepressants, especially the SSRI family which includes Prozac – see page 22.
- There are many others

Many doctors do not discuss these common, potential, unwanted effects with their patients. Presumably they think that they will not take their medication if they believe that it will decrease libido.

Impotence may occur in those who have diabetes mellitus probably because of neurological damage. Many people who suffer from chronic stress also experience impotence. There are a large number of herbs and stress-relieving techniques that can be utilised in these cases.

There are several drugs that have recently come on the market for the treatment of impotence:

Sildenafil (Viagra)

Pfizer released Viagra, the first pharmacological product specifically to treat male impotence, in 1998. Understandably, it received much publicity and later the Nobel Prize was awarded to its discoverers. But by the end of summer of 1998 the first reports were coming in about heart-related deaths in users and many impotent men became anxious about taking it.

It should not be used by men with severe cardiovascular disorders such as unstable angina or severe heart failure (where sexual activity would in any case be contra-indicated), or with drugs prescribed for angina, such as nitrates or amyl nitrate.

Sildenafil has the following unwanted effects (>1%)

- Headache 12.8 per cent
- Flushing 10.4 per cent
- Dizziness 1.2 per cent
- Dyspepsia 4.6 per cent
- Nasal congestion 1.1 per cent
- Altered vision 1.9 per cent, more common at higher doses

- Nosebleeds
- Dyspepsia, more common at higher doses.
- Rarely muscle aches and priapism (persistent erection)

However effective they are, most plant-based medicines will not work unless general lifestyle and dietary considerations are also observed.

Nutrients and general health play an important role in the treatment and prevention of impotence. Some lifestyle issues have a specific role in increasing good health and thereby decreasing the likelihood of sexual inadequacy.

Discussion
The most important first step to overcoming this problem is to discuss it with your partner.

Smoking
Stop smoking – it can lead to impotence for vascular reasons; it narrows blood vessels, reduces blood flow and decreases the strength and duration of an erection.

Diet
Some foods contain sex hormones or may have the ability to influence the levels of sex hormones within your body. They include wheat bran, cruciferous vegetables and legumes. Some spices also help the circulation and may play a part in maintaining the erection process – they include cinnamon, nutmeg and cardamon.

Fat
Large amounts of fat in the diet appear to decrease sex drive in two ways – by causing general lowering of testosterone levels and clogging the arteries so that maintaining an erection is more difficult. Saturated fats are a particular problem – make sure that you have <5 per cent saturated fats per day.

Alcohol
Decrease your alcohol consumption. Alcohol has been known to increase sexual desire but reduce performance since before Shakespeare's time. It is a potent central nervous system depressant and 'brewer's droop' sometimes ensues after several drinks.

Weight
If you are overweight consider losing a few kilos. This can change male hormone levels beneficially and may increase libido.

Exercise
Increasing the amount of exercise that you take per week may also increase libido, general fitness and have anti-fatigue effects.

Coffee
Regular coffee drinkers have been found to be more sexually active than non-drinkers.

Chocolate
Chocolate contains caffeine and also phenyl ethylamine – making it a natural stimulant and anti-depressant. However, avoid products where palm oil and other hydrogenated fat are substituted for cocoa butter.

Bee pollen
Bee pollen contains gonadotrophin, which is similar to a hormone released by the pituitary glands. It activates, stimulates and nourishes the reproductive system. If bee pollen is taken before lovemaking it can reduce fatigue and give you an extra boost.

Zinc
Zinc is necessary for correct functioning of the prostate gland. It is found in large quantities in shellfish including oysters but also in less exotic and expensive foods like pumpkin seeds, eggs, ground mustard, grains and fresh organic fruit and vegetables.

Manganese
This is an important trace mineral. Deficiency states can manifest themselves as sexual indifference. It is best obtained from natural sources such as sunflower seeds, nuts, grains, tropical fruits and beans.

Iodine
Iodine is necessary for optimum thyroid activity required for a good sex drive. Iodine can be taken as iodised salt or as kelp. Certain foods will deplete the thyroid gland – they include members of the *brassica* family such as cabbage, kale and turnips.

Vitamin A
This is required for efficient production of testosterone and maintenance of healthy genitalia in men. In women low levels are often associated with failure to conceive.

Vitamin C
This vitamin is a powerful antioxidant. It is not necessary for sexual potency directly but is needed to keep the testes healthy, so promoting testosterone levels.

Vitamin E
This is essential for the production of sex hormones – it can be taken as a supplement or by eating nuts and seeds.

Glutamine and glutamic acid
These are amino acids that work predominantly as a brain fuel. They appear also to have the ability to improve performance in cases of impotence.

L-Histidine
This is also an amino acid that restores sexual power, reducing impotence and improving orgasm.

Arginine
A supplement of arginine should be taken daily to enhance natural nitric oxide levels, and thereby increase the amount of vasodilators available in the blood. It also increases production of sperm.

Many herbs can be used to improve sexual performance. They have the advantage of having been used for hundreds, maybe thousands, of years and therefore we know their track record – they are perfectly safe even if you have heart disease.

Gotu Cola ~ *Hydrocotyle asiatica*

The aerial parts of this herb are used medicinally. It is considered as both brain food and a rejuvenator, increasing both mental and physical power and strengthens the pituitary gland. It also energises the brain, warding off mental fatigue.

Uses
* Fatigue
* Impotence

Unwanted effects
* Contact allergic dermatitis

Interactions with other herbs
* None

Interactions with other drugs
* None

Contraindications
* Pregnancy and breastfeeding

Recommended dosage:
Dried herb-powdered cotyledons – 3.9g daily
Liquid extract (BPC 1949) 1:1 in 60% alcohol – 2.4ml daily
Tincture (BPC 1934) 1:5 in 60% alcohol – 3-12ml daily

Ashwagandha ~ *Withania somnifera*

The dried root of this herb is mainly used, however the leaves and seeds also have medicinal effects. This plant is also known as Indian Ginseng and has a long history of use in Asian medicine. Ashwagandha is used as a tonic primarily for men, and is said to enhance sex drive and improve erectile function. It also boosts stamina and physical performance. Much research has been carried out into its anti-cancer activity.

Uses

- Impotence
- Adaptogenic
- Analgesic
- Anti-depressant

Unwanted effects

- Nausea
- Dermatitis
- Abdominal pain
- Diarrhoea and vomiting

Interactions with other herbs

- None

Interactions with other drugs

- Barbiturates
- Sedatives
- Anxiolytics

Contraindications

- Pregnancy and breastfeeding

Recommended dosage
Dried root 2-5g daily

Yohimbe ~ *Pausinystalia yohimbe*

This is the bark of an African tree and a powerful sexual stimulant for men. It is a strong aphrodisiac and produces partial or full erections in about 44 to 48 per cent of men. It has been associated with several side effects such as anxiety, flushing, headaches, hallucinations, tachycardia and panic attacks. It should not be taken where there is liver or kidney disease.

Yohimbe has been approved for treatment of impotence of vascular and diabetic origin in the European Community, although it is not currently available in the UK except on prescription from a GP.

In a double blind controlled trial 83 patients were given 10mg of yohimbe three times daily for eight weeks. Yohimbe was found to increase sexual desire, sexual satisfaction, quality of erection and penile rigidity. It was well tolerated.

Yohimbe is also analgesic, raises blood pressure and increases salivary flow.

Uses

- Impotence

Unwanted effects

- Hypertension
- Psychosis
- Auditory effects
- Salivation

Interactions with other herbs

- None

Interactions with other drugs

- Tricyclic antidepressants, such as clomipramine and amitriptyline
- Flupenthixol
- Anti-hypertensive medication
- Alcohol
- Morphine
- Phenothiazines, such as chlorpromazine
- Clonidine
- Barbiturates
- Mono amine oxidase inhibitors
- Beta-blockers
- Sympathomimetics
- Naloxone

Contraindications

- Psychosis
- Parkinson's disease
- Depression
- Anxiety/panic attacks
- High blood pressure
- Kidney disease
- Pregnancy and breastfeeding
- Liver disease
- Chronic inflammation of the genitals
- Allergic hypersensitivity
- Cardiac disease

Recommended dosage

Non-organic erectile dysfunction:
Capsules (yohimbine hydrochloride) – 10mg three times daily

Erectile impotence:
Capsules – 5.4mg three times daily

Puncture Vine Fruit ~ *Tribulus terrestris*

This herb is an anti-depressant, bodybuilding tonic, fertility enhancer and aphrodisiac herb used mainly by men. It has a long and interesting history. It appears in the great medical treatise, the *Charaka Samhita* of 700BC, so probably has one of the longest documented clinical usages of any herb known to man and certainly longer than any drug you care to name.

Uses

- Impotence

Unwanted effects
- None

Interactions with other herbs
- None

Interactions with other drugs
- None

Contraindications
- None

Recommended dosage

Tea	5-10ml herb
Capsules	1-3 daily

Quebracho ~ *Aspidosperma quebracho-blanco*

The bark of this tree is used medicinally and is considered a male aphrodisiac in South America. It is native to Chile, Argentina, south east Bolivia and south east Brazil. It contains the compound, yohimbe.

Quebracho is also used for chronic respiratory problems because it stimulates the respiratory centres and is an expectorant.

Uses
- Impotence

Unwanted effects
- Nausea (with large doses)

Interactions with other herbs
- None

Interactions with other drugs
- None

Contraindications
- High blood pressure
- Dizziness

Recommended dosage
A single dose of 1–2g of the plant

Damiana ~ *Turnera aphrodisiaca*

This herb has traditionally been used to arouse sexual desires in either sex. The medicinal parts are the leaves, which are harvested during the flowering season. Damiana grows mainly in the region of the Gulf of Mexico, the Caribbean and southern Africa.

It was available in the USA in the 1870s as a tincture and used as an aphrodisiac to 'improve the sexual ability of the enfeebled and aged'. It may increase pelvic blood supply and secretions.

Uses
- Impotence

Unwanted effects
- Irritation of urethral mucosa
- Hepatic dysfunction
- Hallucinations

Interactions with other herbs
- None

Interactions with other drugs
- Anti-diabetic medications

Contraindications
- Pregnancy and breastfeeding

Recommended dosage
Dried herb   2-4g three times daily
Tincture   up to 2.5ml three times daily

Muira Puama ~ *Iriosma ovata*

The bark and roots of this herb is used in South America as a sexual rejuvenator and is very highly regarded. It appears to work in both sexes.

In a study in France over 250 men who experienced impotence and low libido were asked to take muira puama daily for two weeks. Sixty-two per cent claimed an improvement in sexual performance and increased libido.

In a further study of 94 men with impotence and loss of body strength, 55 per cent reported restored sexual function and 66 per cent increased frequency of sexual encounters.

Uses
- Loss of libido
- Impotence

Unwanted effects
- None

Interactions with other herbs
- None

Interactions with other drugs
- None

Contraindications
Pregnancy and breastfeeding

Recommended dosage
Tea   made of 5-10g herb
Capsules   1-3 daily

Oats ~ *Avena sativa*

I make no excuses for mentioning oats again (see also pages 54 and 78). They have been used as a medicine all over the world mainly to restore sex drive and generally give more energy. There are a number of steroid-like substances in oats that displace testosterone from sex hormone-binding globulin and allow more 'real' testosterone to remain free and active in the bloodstream. This results in a boost to sex lives, as well as increasing motivation and energy levels.

Uses
• Low libido
• Exhaustion

Ginseng ~ *Panax ginseng/Panax quinquefolium*

Ginseng is known to strengthen sexual activity. This herb is an adaptogen. Panax ginseng has been shown to improve physical and mental performance and have anti-fatigue effects. It has already been discussed on page 73.

Uses
• Low libido

St John's Wort ~ *Hypericum perforatum*

This has no traditional use as an aphrodisiac but where there is a neurogenic reason for impotence such as diabetes it may increase nerve impulses to the penis, thus resolving the problem. It has been discussed in some detail on page 47.

Uses

• Impotence

• Mild to moderate depression

• Fatigue

Ginkgo ~ *Gingko biloba*

This herb is known to increase blood flow to the brain. It has no traditional use as an aphrodisiac, being more commonly prescribed for intermittent claudication and cognitive dysfunction. But as it increases blood flow to the small capillaries of the penis it helps in vascular causes of impotence. Several people have noticed that ginkgo has produced an increase in the intensity and length of orgasm (in both men and women) It has already been discussed as a treatment for PMS – see page 196.

Uses

• Impotence

• Cognitive dysfunction

19 | Diet

The health of the people is the highest law (Salus populi suprema lex).

~ Cicero

Many of you may not realise the effect of your diet on the development and cure of your cancer. I regret to say that, all too often, patients get no useful advice on this subject at all.

There has never been a more important time to eat well than during your recovery from cancer so please take time to read this chapter and consider its relevance in terms of what *you* eat. I am aware that some people may need to change how they live and probably stop eating and drinking products that they enjoy.

In the 50 plus years since the end of the last war, UK farming has become industrialised, encouraged by the government and our membership of the European community. The European Common Agricultural Policy makes payment to farmers based on, not the *quality*, but the *quantity* of produce. In response to this farmers have increased production dramatically, often generating huge surpluses, hence the notorious 'grain mountains' and 'wine lakes' of the last decades.

This industrial production has necessitated the use of synthetic fertilisers, pesticides, animal drugs, antibiotics and hormones. We have adopted the practice of using unnatural feeds for animals and factory farming on a much larger scale than the rest of Europe. In addition to altering the nature of the food we eat these methods have promoted wholesale environmental damage, animal welfare issues, pollution of water sources, loss of habitat for native species, including loss of hedgerows and damage to soil structure.

There has been a move away from traditional farming practices that use many different species often in rotation, towards practices using very limited or single species (mono-culture). At one time almost every county had its own particular breed of cattle. These were suited to the local environment and conditions, each vigorously producing meat with varied tastes and textures. Now throughout Europe the predominant breed of cattle is derived from modified Holstein stock, providing a compromise animal in an attempt to meet all types of conditions with maximum yield. Because of the limited gene pool, these animals are gravely at risk of infectious diseases which could sweep through stock with devastating effects, therefore chemical supplements and antibiotics are used widely in order to maintain meat and milk production. Cows are given hormones to increase milk yield. Much of the milk and dairy products that we drink contain the hormones and antibiotics excreted in the cow's milk.

Many animals are being fed on imported genetically modified (GM) crops and so much of the meat, eggs, poultry, farmed fish we eat and the milk we drink *may* be coming from animals fed a GM diet. There is no obligation to declare this on products at present. Some supermarkets do plan to phase out GM feeds in their own-brand labels.

In 1999 GM companies tried to introduce their products into the marketplace – there was a public outcry and retailers were forced to declare whether their products contained GM ingredients. We have no idea what effect these products will have on our health. In nature genes NEVER cross the species barrier – now, in the laboratory, this is being done without full understanding of its long-term consequences. It is possible that virulent new drug resistant bacteria or even new diseases will develop.

If new genes are put into plants could this trigger respiratory or inflammatory reactions in the one to two per cent of the population who suffer from food allergies? Or skin reactions in those who handle them? What ecological changes will these new species bring about? Will theses changes affect our health? Will they increase or decrease our susceptibility to cancer? Clearly at present there are many more questions than answers.

In the 1980s there were widespread moves towards food irradiation. This technique was backed by the government and food industry, despite its health implications. There was widespread public opposition because it was generally believed that it encouraged sloppy hygiene. Workers might think 'It's being irradiated so what does it matter?' It might disguise food that was otherwise unfit for human consumption; and it might kill off most of the beneficial bacteria but only some of the harmful ones.

Irradiation is also known to decrease vitamin content of fresh fruit and vegetables by up to 90 per cent. Public opinion won the day and it was stopped, only to be quietly re-introduced about a year later through European legislation.

PCBs (polychlorinated biphenyls) have been found in our food – they are subtle toxins that accumulate in our fat. They are also hormone mimics and are excreted in breast milk in sufficient quantities to cause immune, thyroid and clotting disorders in babies. PCBs have been implicated in the development of cancers. In Belgium, in the wake of a food scandal in 1999, tests on 20,000 food samples showed a four per cent rate of contamination, it is estimated that this will cause up to 8300 extra cases of cancer.

PCBs are clearly undesirable, but in the UK we are not even monitoring their effects and concentration. In 2001, PCBs were found in high levels in eggs from a farm in Anglesey by accident. Inspectors were actually checking for dioxin fallout from the pyres burnt to destroy animals slaughtered in the foot and mouth outbreak. PCBs, formerly used in the plastics industry, have not been made since the 1980s but have accumulated in fish in the North Sea. We feed North Sea fish meal to animals and so this tainted feed contaminates the meat, eggs and other meat products that we eat.

Politicians and food producers seem unaware that these dietary issues are having a profound effect on our health as a nation. There is now little doubt about the links between cancer and what we eat – estimates vary but at least 75 per cent of cancers are due to dietary and lifestyle factors which include smoking, alcohol consumption, hormonal imbalances, radiation exposure, food additives, drugs and infections.

Trying to collate all available studies is a gargantuan task and the minute that an article or book is written it is probably out of date. Between 1983 and 1993 there have been a staggering 5000 mainstream studies about nutrition in cancer. In the year following that over 500 more studies were published.

There is no doubt that your best defence against cancer or armoury in the recovery from cancer is a strong nutritional offensive. I have compiled general guidelines for all cancer patients and also some general recommendations for specific problems.

Generally food consists of

A. MACRONUTRIENTS – these make up the majority of what we eat:

Carbohydrates

Basically these break down to sugar during the process of digestion. They include all sweets such as chocolate, cakes and biscuits as well as stodgy foods such as pasta, potatoes, bread and also foods containing other types of sugars such as milk, vegetables and fruit. They provide the body with energy, not only for physical activity, but also for the body's own metabolic processes which will need to be accelerated during healing. If you eat excess carbohydrates, they will be converted to cholesterol or fat in the body.

Proteins

These include essential amino acids used to build and repair the body. It stands to reason that those with the highest requirements are children, adolescents and pregnant women. But any illness necessitating cell repair and the regulation of metabolism will also require additional resources. Protein is found in meat, fish and eggs and also in pulses, grains, nuts and seeds.

Fats

This comprises visible fat on meat etc but also include essential fatty acids. They provide essential building materials for the body. Cell membranes and nerves require fats to function correctly as does the blood clotting mechanism, the production of hormones and anti-inflammatory chemicals in the body. They are also used as a source of energy.

B. MICRONUTRIENTS – these are no less important but are taken into the body in lesser quantities

1. ***Other naturally occurring chemicals with powerful anti-cancer properties***

These include beta carotene, quercetin, indoles, isothiocyanates and omega 3 fatty acids.

2. *Vitamins* (Adults)

Official recommended doses. The figures in this table apply to people 19-50+ years.

Vitamin	RDA EC	RNI UK	Sources
Vitamin A★ (retinol and beta-carotene)	800µg	700µg	Retinol: liver, eggs, butter. Beta-carotene: carrots, tomatoes, broccoli, spinach, apricots.
Vitamin B1 (thiamine)	1.4mg	1.0mg	Eggs, brown rice, barley, pork.
Vitamin B2 (riboflavine)	1.6mg	1.3mg	Green leafy vegetables, eggs, bread, cereal, fish.
Vitamin B3 (niacin)	18mg	17mg	Meat, fish, cereals, eggs.
Vitamin B5 (pantothenic acid) ø	6mg	3-7mg	Wholegrain cereals, brown rice, molasses, eggs, yeast, liver and kidneys.
Vitamin B6 (pyridoxine)	2mg	1.4mg	Vegetables, wholegrain cereals, fish, meat, eggs.
Folic acid	200µg	200µg	Nuts, green leafy vegetables, eggs, wheat germ, bananas, oranges, liver and kidney.
Vitamin B12 (cobalamin)	1.0µg	1.5µg	Liver, beef, pork, eggs, fish.
Vitamin C (ascorbic acid)	60mg	40mg	All fresh fruits and vegetables, especially citric fruits, kiwi fruits, blackcurrant and broccoli.
Vitamin D★	5µg	10µg (over 65)	Eggs, butter, oily fish, fish liver oil.
Vitamin E★ ø	10mg	>4mg	Green leafy vegetables, wholegrains, peanuts, eggs, broccoli, wheat germ, soya beans, olive oil.
Biotin ø	150µg	10-200µg	Nuts, fruit, beef liver, egg yolk, kidneys, brown rice, brewer's yeast.
Vitamin K★ ø		70µg	Green leafy vegetables, soya bean oils and margarines, milk, liver and kidney.

★denotes a fat soluble vitamin – others are water soluble

RDA denotes recommended daily allowance (blanks denote there is no recommended amount.)

RNI denotes Reference Nutrient Intake defined as an amount of nutrient that is enough, or more than enough, for approx. 97 per cent of people.

Fruit and vegetables soon lose their vitamin content when transported and stored. For instance an orange may contain 180mg of vitamin C or none at all! Where possible buy local fruit and vegetables in season rather than those shipped from the other side of the world.

3. *Minerals* including trace elements

Mineral	RDA EC	RNI UK	Sources
Boron *			Water, fruits, vegetables, nuts and seeds, wine and beer.
Calcium	800mg	700mg	Hard water, yoghurt, fish, eggs, liver and kidney, wholegrain cereals, pulses, green leafy vegetables, dates, nuts.
Chloride		2500mg	Table salt and salt substitutes, vegetables, meat.
Chromium		25µg	Liver and kidney, whole grain cereals, yeast.
Copper		1.2mg	Fish, liver and kidneys, green leafy vegetables, nuts, mushrooms, avocados, seaweed, cocoa.
Iodine	150µg	140µg	Fish, shellfish, meat, liver and kidney, wholegrain cereals, peanuts, green leafy vegetables, seaweed, pineapple, grapes, iodised salt.
Iron	14mg	14.8(F)mg 8.7(M)mg	Egg yolks, liver and kidney, red meat, green leafy vegetables, cocoa, shellfish, wholegrain cereals, seaweed, dates, figs, nuts and seeds.
Magnesium	300mg	300mg	Fish, shellfish, whole grain cereals, green leafy vegetables, mushrooms, seaweed, hard water, cocoa, nuts and seeds.
Manganese ø		1.4mg	Wholegrain cereals, pineapple, green leafy vegetables, garlic, carrots, potatoes, sunflower seeds, tea, root ginger
Molybdenum ø		50-400µg	Buckwheat, beans, wholegrains, wheatgerm, soya beans, liver, meat, eggs, vegetables

Mineral	RDA EC	RNI UK	Sources
Phosphorus	800mg	550mg	Meat, liver and kidney, fish, chicken, wholegrain rice, pulses, cabbage, mushrooms, seaweed, dates and figs, seeds.
Potassium		3500mg	Pulses, fruit, wholegrain rice and cereals, nuts and seeds, cocoa, LoSalt.
Sodium		1600mg	Table salt, meat, vegetables.
Selenium		75µg	Egg yolk, fish, liver and kidney, cabbage, mushrooms, garlic, wheatgerm.
Silica Δ			Water, fruit and vegetables.
Sulphur Δ			Fish, meat, wholegrain cereals, pulses, garlic.
Vanadium ✷			Eggs, fish, shellfish, liver and kidney, wholegrain cereals, wholegrain rice, pulses, cabbage, carrots, mushrooms, garlic, seaweed, sprouted seeds, sunflower seeds, olive oil.
Zinc	15mg	7.0(f)mg 9.5(m)mg	Eggs, meat, shellfish, liver and kidney, wholegrain cereals, pulses, carrots, potatoes, garlic, seaweed, sprouted seeds, seeds, tea, root ginger.

ø There is no UK RNI for these but the Panel on Dietary Reference Values of the Committee on Medical Aspects of Food Policy suggest the values as safe intakes.

Δ These are essential trace elements but are found in so many different foods that deficiency is not considered to be a possibility.

✷ These are not considered to be essential trace minerals but are present in all diets.

It has been estimated that mineral levels have been reduced in fruit and vegetables by 76 per cent in the last 20 years. This is because:

- Our land is being over-farmed and soil gradually loses its mineral content unless it is replaced by the addition of mineral-rich manure. Many of the minerals necessary for our health are not needed to make plants grow so the farming community does not find it financially beneficial to add them to the land. Instead only those minerals needed to make the plants grow (nitrogen, phosphate and potassium) are used as fertilisers.

- Refining food removes minerals. Ninety per cent of minerals are refined out of rice, white flour and white sugar.
- We need more minerals to counteract the effects of pollution.

Nutritional recommendations

Shopping

Shop regularly and buy the best that you can afford. Avoid damaged, stale and wilted foods as these are more likely to contain carcinogens (cancer-causing substances) and less likely to contain vitamins. Avoid irradiated fruit and vegetables where possible.

Try to stop buying and eating processed foods. This includes anything that comes in cans, boxes or packets. Aim for as wide a variety of foods as possible over each seven to 10 day period.

If you must buy processed foods, cook-chill foods, ready meals, etc, look for those labelled with '100 per cent organic ingredients'. Be aware that these will NEVER be an adequate substitute for home cooked foods and should only ever be used occasionally. They are prepared on an industrial scale and often contain ingredients that would not be acceptable to you in your own kitchen. These ingredients are added to compensate for loss of flavour and altered consistency of the product and to extend shelf life. Examples are monosodium glutamate, milk powder, caramel, sodium caseinate, and hydrogenated vegetable oils.

Be wary of foods labelled low fat. These contain more additives than the full fat versions, and more sugar to compensate for loss of taste – but excess sugar is converted to fat in the body!

Eat wholegrains, lentils beans, nuts, seeds, fresh fruit and vegetables. Avoid refined, white or overcooked food and eat four or more servings a day of wholegrains such as rye, millet, rice, oats, wholewheat, corn, quinoa as cereals, breads, pasta or pulses.

Vegetables and Fruit

These top the list of anti-cancer foods. They are a rich source of cancer-preventing vitamins A and C and beta carotene. Reduce refined and over-cooked food, including over-cooked vegetables that will have lost a majority of their vitamins. Stir-frying or steaming is a good way of preserving nutrients.

CANCER: HERBS IN HOLISTIC HEALTHCARE

Make sure that you eat five helpings of fruit or vegetables daily not including potatoes. Half of these should be raw. Eat an orange-coloured vegetable or fruit every day. Some people find this difficult but it is well worth trying and can be achieved with a little planning.

Buy fresh vegetables and fruit, preferably organic, regularly – at least twice per week. The ultimate ideal is to grow your own fruit and vegetables if possible. All deteriorate rapidly in terms of vitamin content after picking. Look for the logo of the UK Soil Association or the Biodynamic Agricultural Association, or visit your local Women's Institute Market or Farmers' Market for locally grown organic produce.

Start the day by having fresh or dried fruit for breakfast perhaps added to porridge, or you could add a cooked tomato or mushrooms to a hot breakfast. A glass of fresh orange juice also counts as a portion. Fruit is also a useful mid-morning snack or can be eaten at lunchtime with a salad or salad sandwich. Vegetables, beans or salad can be the central part of your main meal either in stir-fries, steamed, or in a casserole.

All vegetables are beneficial but some are more beneficial than others! Foods with the highest anti-cancer activity include garlic, soya beans, cabbage, ginger, liquorice and umbelliferous vegetables such as fennel.

Beta carotene is the nutrient which supplies the deep orange colour in carrots, red/orange peppers, mangoes, cantaloupe melon. Some dark green vegetables such as broccoli also contain significant amounts of beta carotene. It has been found to destroy human cancer cells in several ways. It is especially effective against lung cancer (see page 266).

In a review of 20 studies on allium-containing vegetables (onions, garlic, leeks, etc) and their influence on cancer, a protective effect was shown without a single exception. They contain the powerful natural anti-cancer chemical – quercitin. The colon and other parts of the gastro-intestinal tract were particularly protected, confirmed by the Iowa Health Study of 1994, which included 41,000 women aged 55-69.

Garlic was particularly beneficial – in one laboratory study a garlic compound, ajoene, was shown to be toxic to malignant cells. In the USA researchers found that garlic boosted the anti-cancer action of white blood cells in the laboratory though whether this also applies in human subjects remains to be seen.

Tomatoes are high in the natural chemical lycopene. This can have powerful effects in preventing cancers, especially of the bladder and prostate gland. Watermelon also contains large quantities of lycopene; and there is a small amount in apricots.

Cruciferous vegetables can lower the risk of colon cancer. They contain indoles and isothiocyanates that help reduce and prevent certain cancers. Many are also high in beta carotene. Two tablespoons of cooked cabbage daily has also been found to help prevent stomach cancer.

- Cabbage-all types
- Brussels sprouts
- Bok choy
- Cauliflower
- Rutabaga

- Spring greens
- Kale
- Broccoli
- Horseradish
- Kohlrabi

Citrus fruits (grapefruit, oranges, mandarins, lemons, etc) contain vitamin C and also folic acid, potassium, pectin and over 60 flavonoids. These have a wide variety of actions including anti-inflammatory and anti-cancer activity, especially regarding cancer of the oesophagus.

Celery seeds contain a natural chemical that stimulates an enzyme called glutathione S-transferase, thought to be an inhibitor of cancer cells. Similar chemicals are found in garlic and onion, broccoli and other cruciferous vegetables, and ginger and turmeric.

If you don't feel like eating fruit and vegetables, why not juice them or make some soup? This makes them easier to digest and assimilate.

Meat

Consumption of *lean* red meat is not a risk factor for cancer according to a study of 3,660 men and women in the UK. Buy whole unprocessed pieces of meat rather than sausages, rissoles, meat pies and burgers that may contain MRM (mechanically recovered meat from the bones) or Proticon meat (mechanically recovered from crushed bones). These are potential vectors of disease-causing agents. Buying organic meat from a reputable source will reduce the amount of unwanted chemicals taken in through the diet.

Don't buy processed meat products such as nuggets, pates, spreads, luncheon meat, knockwurst or frankfurters. They usually contain high levels of nitrites which can interact with natural chemicals in our food to form nitrosamines – potent cancer-causing agents. They also reduce the vitamin A content of foods.

Don't eat overcooked meat or burnt fat. Smoked foods such as fish or bacon may also carry the same risk. Consumption of these products may predispose to the development of stomach cancer.

Cooking

Reappraise your cooking methods. Change frying, barbecuing, microwaving and re-heating for baking, steaming, grilling and stir-frying.

Nuts and Seeds

Sesame and sunflowers seeds are rich in vitamin E, selenium, calcium and zinc. Eat a spoonful every day to keep antioxidant levels high.

Fats and Oils

Decrease your consumption of saturated fats – this is basically animal fat; such as fat on meat, suet, lard, dripping and cream. Research has shown a link between these and heart disease and some cancers but they are only dangerous if eaten to excess. They are natural, not damaged by processing, and have co-existed with us in nature for a long time. Our body needs to use them as fuel and as an ingredient in cell structure. Aim for less than 5 per cent of saturated fat in your diet.

It is also essential that you eat some types of essential fatty acids in order to produce natural anti-inflammatory agents, well-balanced hormone profiles, healthy skin, and so on.

Minimise consumption of palm and coconut oils as these contain a high proportion of saturated fats.

You need to eat some types of fats for a healthy metabolism. One of these essential fatty acids is fish oil. Consume oily fish regularly, two to five times per week, or take a fish oil supplement derived from fish from cool, clean northern oceans. This should be high in omega 3 fatty acids. It is adviseable to take a supplement of vitamin E to prevent oxidation of this oil.

In animal experiments fish oil retarded tumour growth in numerous studies and epidemiological studies showed that men who eat oily fish or took a fish oil supplement had reduced levels of colon cancer. There are also some promising results in studies of breast cancer patients. Fish oil has also been shown to lower HDL cholesterol. It is also known to promote production of natural anti-inflammatory agents within the body, which is naturally beneficial to patients with arthritis and other inflammatory conditions such as fibromyalgia.

Add a variety of fresh nuts (unsalted) and seeds to your diet regularly. They are high in fibre, mono-unsaturated (essential fatty acids) fats and selenium (you require 200mcg of selenium daily or three Brazil nuts). Selenium is necessary to maintain normal hormone function and may have a role in cancer prevention. Nuts and seeds are also thought to promote a healthy heart. They can be added to muesli, salads and rice dishes or eaten as a snack.

Other essential fatty acids include oil of evening primrose, linseed oil and hemp seed oil. Deficiency of these will affect cells and tissues throughout the entire body and adversely affect many metabolic processes and homeostatic mechanisms. These include kidney malfunctions and fluid retention; immune dysfunction; tissue and joint inflammation; hypertension; high blood fats; muscle weakness; dry eyes, mouth and skin.

We need to take in a combination. Some experts say that we need a ratio of 2:1 of Omega 3s (α-linoleic acid – found in flax seed [also known as linseed] hemp seed, canola , soya bean, walnut and dark green leaves, and eicosapentaenoic acid (found in the oils of cold water fish) compared to Omega 6s (linoleic acid – found in sunflower, hemp seed, soya bean, walnut, pumpkin, sesame and flax oils and γ-linolenic acid – found in borage, blackcurrant seed oils and oil of evening primrose).

Replace margarine with butter. Margarine is highly processed and contains many undesirable chemicals. It is high in trans fatty acids, now known to be harmful to health, and may encourage the growth of some types of cancer such as breast cancer (see page 261). Butter is a natural product, but like all foodstuffs it can be contaminated, so choose one from a clean environment where environmental pollution is less and eat it sparingly.

Avoid hydrogenated fats. These are known to adversely affect the immune system, interfere with liver enzymes necessary for detoxification, make platelets more sticky, raise cholesterol levels and interfere with cell membrane function and permeability.

Hydrogenated fats are found in:

- Cakes
- Biscuits
- Chocolate bars
- Breakfast cereals

- Peanut butter
- Instant soups
- Cream crackers
- Crisps

Frying is not recommended, either shallow or deep. The heat which results alters the chemical structure of the oil or fat used, making it even more dangerous to health than it was formerly. The least damaging oils seem to be coconut, palm, palm kernel, cocoa butter and butter. Never allow oils to smoke and never 'burn' food. If you must fry anything throw the fat away afterwards as it will have an altered chemical structure.

In commercial deep-frying operations the same batch of oil is kept at high temperature for days. Many altered molecules are found in such fats and we can be pretty sure that they do not improve our health. Recent research has identified cancer-containing molecules in chips, crisps and other fried snack foods.

Use only best quality olive oil – buy this regularly keep it in a cool dark place in glass containers.

Carageenan

Avoid products containing the food additive carageenan. This is synthesised from seaweed but has long been implicated in causing inflammatory conditions in the bowel and recently in causing breast cancer. It is used as a thickening agent by the food industry and is found in a variety of goods such as yoghurts, ice cream, cheeses, processed puddings and toothpaste.

Sugars

Cut sugar out of your diet as much as possible. It doesn't matter if it is white sugar, brown sugar, honey, maple syrup, rice syrup, corn syrup or any similar sweetener. After digestion and assimilation sugar is turned into hard fats within the body. Consequently, among other adverse effects on health, it makes platelets more sticky, interferes with insulin function and the function of essential fatty acids. Most of us are aware that sugar also damages teeth, as well as being a food source for fungi, yeasts and cancer cells. It interferes with vitamin C transport; increases adrenaline function making it a powerful internal stressor; cross-links proteins and speeds the ageing process; and leeches important minerals from the body, most notably calcium and chromium.

Colourants and Sweeteners
Avoid added colourants such as red food dye. These are thought to cause health problems.

Avoid artificial sweeteners such as aspartame. They degrade in the body to chemicals that may be toxic to some people. Of 6000 complaints received by the Food & Drug Administration (FDA) in the USA, from 1985-1988, 80 per cent concerned aspartame. This is found in diet drinks, low calorie foods and is substituted for sugar in many foods.

Fluids
Drink plenty of bottled water (two litres per day). You can also drink organic fruit juices if you like them.

Restrict consumption of alcohol and fizzy drinks. High alcohol intake has been associated with cancer of the mouth, tongue, oesophagus and liver.

Cut out all caffeine-containing products such as tea, coffee and chocolate. If you can't stop completely reduce these as much as possible. Very high levels of caffeine – that is nine or more drinks per day – have been linked to the development of a range of cancers including pancreatic, kidney and ovarian.

Herbs and Spices
If you don't already include fresh herbs in your diet – add some! Herbs that belong to the family *Labiatae* such as basil, mint, oregano, sage, rosemary and thyme, are known to have strong antioxidant/anti-cancer activity. They are now readily available at most supermarkets but also easy to grow in your garden or even a window box.

Don't buy irradiated herbs, fruit and vegetables. Irradiation kills beneficial bacteria as well as harmful ones. It causes loss of up to 90 per cent of vitamins.

Some spices also have a powerful antioxidant effect and bring many benefits to the health of those who eat them regularly. Asian patients in the

Leicester area have a far lower risk of cancer in general than other ethnic groups. Research is going on into possible dietary reasons for this and so far a high intake of the spice turmeric appears to be the most likely cause.

Fibre

Ensure that you eat sufficient fibre (>30g) in your diet every day. There is no universally effective way of achieving this. A high intake of fruit and vegetables, nuts and seeds, pulses and other high fibre products will help. If you can, increase your consumption of wholemeal bread, wholemeal pasta and brown rice while reducing the amount of white flour, white pasta, white rice and white sugar.

Eggs

Don't be afraid to eat eggs. Evidence points to their benefits rather than any harmful effects. In America, following advice from the American Heart Association consumption of eggs fell in the 1990s to half of what it was in 1945. However, there was no corresponding decline in heart disease, in fact it continued to rise! Modern research has shown that eggs have the perfect balance of proteins for humans, assisting the healing process. In addition, the lecithin that they contain aids fat assimilation and raises the beneficial portion of cholesterol (HDL). Obviously free range eggs are the most helpful to health.

Milk

Eliminate milk and milk products from your diet completely. There is now increasing evidence that we are consuming increasing amounts of hormones and growth factors in our diet. These are found in dairy products because they are fed to cattle and dairy herds with the aim of increasing meat and milk yields. Cows are milked even when pregnant, further increasing the amount of oestrogen in the milk. Other undesirable chemicals, such as dioxin, are also found in milk. Diets high in dairy produce have been linked to the development of breast and prostate cancer. There are plenty of other sources of calcium in your diet including fish, green vegetables and water!

Weight

Keep your weight within the normal range for your height (see also page 171). Obesity may increase your risk of some cancers – even being only five per cent overweight increases your risk of developing cancer of the breast, gallbladder or uterus.

Exercise

Take regular exercise. If you can, go for a walk or do some other exercise for 20 minutes three times per week. Researchers have concluded that there is a definite link between lack of physical activity and colon and breast cancers and a possible link between lack of activity and development of prostate cancer. Lung and uterine cancers show a possible link and testicular and ovarian cancers show little or no correlation.

Selenium

Low levels of the mineral selenium may be relevant to the development of an increasing number of cancers, in particular breast and colon cancer. In general, nowadays, vegetables have lower levels of this and many other minerals because modern farming methods only replace certain chemicals into the soil. In some European countries it is compulsory for farmers to add a selenium supplement to the land, but not in the UK. In north east Scotland, an area known for low selenium levels, there are high rates of colon cancer.

Multivitamin and mineral supplements

Consider taking a multivitamin and mineral supplement if you feel your diet may be deficient in essential minerals and vitamins. American research has found that low levels of zinc in the blood have been associated with certain cancers, most notably head and neck cancers, but also prostate cancer. Zinc is also necessary to maintain a healthy immune system.

It has been discovered that wherever soil concentration of iodine is lowest then the level of cancer is higher. This applies especially to the oestrogen-dependent cancers (breast, uterus).

For example, the oral contraceptive depletes the body of some vitamins so women taking this should supplement with vitamins B2, B6, B12 and C, and folic acid.

The body can only synthesise two vitamins: vitamin D, which is produced when the skin is exposed to ultra-violet radiation, and vitamin K, made by bacteria in the large intestine. All other vitamins must be taken into the body regularly. Only the fat-soluble vitamins (A, D, E and K) can be stored and a deficiency may not be apparent for a year.

When choosing a supplement don't overdo it – vitamins and minerals are only needed in small amounts. Too much may actually be harmful so pay attention to the recommended daily allowance (RDA). Some, such as vitamin C, are water-soluble so excess is not stored in the body but is excreted in the urine. Others are fat-soluble and the body will attempt to store excess with possible harmful effects.

Many vitamins are now known to be associated with lowering the risk of certain cancers. Vitamin A may play a part in preventing cancers of the throat, oesophagus, lung, stomach, large bowel, bladder and prostate gland. Vitamin C is associated with a lowering risk of cancer of the oesophagus, breast, cervix, bladder, stomach, skin, lung, colon, mouth and pancreas. Vitamin E may generally reduce the risk of developing cancer by protecting fats from going rancid – this is associated with generally higher levels of carcinogens. Vitamin B6 may reduce the risk of cancer of cervix and bladder.

In summary: vitamin A, beta carotene, vitamin C, vitamin E and selenium are important nutrients in the fight against cancer.

In the last 20 years much research has been carried out into the effects of certain foods on various cancers:

Breast cancer

Breast cancer remains one of the commonest cancers in women – there will be 38,000 new cases each year (200 of them are men) and 13,000 will die per annum. Between one in eight and one in 2500 women are affected, depending on age and where they live. It is the commonest cause of death in women between 45 and 55 years. The UK has the highest incidence of breast cancer in the world and has a high mortality, but 74 per cent survive for more than five years.

Breast cancer is most likely to be discovered after the menopause but a substantial number of women are affected beforehand or even in their teens. It has recently been overtaken by lung cancer as the most common cancer in women.

Flaxseed (linseed) is a very rich source of lignans, which appear to be anti-carcinogenic. They are known to produce metabolites that are structurally similar to oestrogens and can bind to oestrogen receptors and inhibit growth of oestrogen-sensitive tumours such as breast and uterine cancers. Taking a teaspoon of linseeds or a linseed oil supplement daily would seem a sensible precaution. An Australian study involving 144 breast cancer patients and controls showed that increased excretion of lignan metabolites was associated with tumour regression.

A diet high in natural plant chemicals such as phyto-oestrogens may play a part in reducing the risk of breast cancer. In areas of Asia where the diet is high in soya beans – which in turn are high in phyto-oestrogens – breast cancer rates are among the lowest in the world.

Taking a supplement of fish oil or eating oily fish two to five times per week has shown some promising results in preventing recurrence of breast cancer.

Eating polyunsaturated fats found in some vegetable oils can increase breast cancer risk by 69 per cent. However, the most favourable are olive oils and canola oil, which can decrease risk by up to 45 per cent. Many oils sold as 'healthy' such as sunflower and safflower, could be damaging your health because they are processed using very high heat that changes their chemical structure making them potentially dangerous. It is important to use *only* a good quality virgin olive oil that should be stored in an opaque glass bottle, kept cool and out of the light.

Fat in the diet has long been suspected as a culprit in the development of breast cancer, but studies give conflicting results. A French study confirmed an increased risk with higher consumption of saturated fat but the Harvard Nurses Study did not. Japanese women with their traditional low fat diet also have low incidence of breast cancer but catch up if they emigrate into a Western culture.

I believe that drinking milk and milk-products is the cause. Japanese diet has NO milk products at all, whereas communities with a high incidence of breast cancer also have a high consumption of dairy products. In a Norwegian study of over 25,000 women, those who consumed three glasses of milk daily had three times the risk of developing breast cancer than those who drank half a cup or less. This was confirmed by a Japanese study carried out in the laboratory on rats that found that milk, yoghurt and margarine promoted growth of breast tumours.

Eliminate milk and milk products from your diet. There is now increasing evidence that we are eating increasing amounts of hormones, particularly IGF-1 oestrogen and growth factors, particularly bGH- bovine growth hormone, in our diet. These are found in dairy products because they are fed to cattle and dairy herds to increase meat and milk yields.

In an Italian study of 5000 women it was deduced that breast cancer rates increase with higher intakes of bread and cereal dishes, sugar and pork meat, and decreased with the intake of olive oil, raw vegetables, fish, vitamin E and beta carotene-containing fruit and vegetables.

If you already have been diagnosed with breast cancer then coenzyme Q10 (90-1200mg daily) together with antioxidants and essential fatty acids have been successful in the treatment and secondary prevention of this disease.

Lung cancer

Lung cancer is the most common cancer in the UK. Since research conducted by Sir Richard Doll there has been no doubt that the main causative factor is inhaling tobacco smoke, either actively or passively. Additional causes include occupational exposure to asbestos, nickel, radon and chromium – 38,500 people are affected per year; 24,000 are men. There is a 5 per cent survival rate.

However, there is also some evidence that vegetables offer protective effects, especially yellow/orange varieties high in beta carotene such as carrots, apricots, red or orange peppers, tomatoes, etc (see below). This is because of their high antioxidant effects. It has also been noted that in Japan, where smoking levels are very high, lung cancer levels are low. Recent research has pointed to the anti-cancer properties of green tea. Foods high in beta carotene are:

- Apricots
- Peaches
- Sweet potatoes
- Carrots
- Spinach
- Pumpkin
- Cantaloupe melon
- Beet greens

- Vegetable squash
- Pink grapefruit
- Mango
- Green lettuces
- Broccoli
- Brussels sprouts
- Savoy cabbage

Colo-rectal or large bowel cancer

This is the fourth commonest form of cancer worldwide, accounting for 10 per cent of all cancers. In the UK it is the third commonest cause of cancer – 34,000 new cases are diagnosed per year and it is the second greatest cause of death at 14,600 per year. Global deaths from this form of cancer are on the increase, especially in the industrialised nations. It is the second commonest cause of death from cancer in the EU, with a 40 per cent survival rate.

This is a form of cancer where risk is *definitely* modified by diet. Alcohol and diets high in meat increase the risk. The incidence of colorectal cancers in people who eat a lot of processed meats such as sausages, bacon, etc, is high; red meat, has been shown to be insignificant. Diets high in sugar and animal fats may also increase risk as does a family history of colon cancer, a history of ulcerative colitis and/or polyps in the gut, or infestation by *Schistosoma sinesis*. Obesity and smoking also increase the risk of developing this form of cancer.

Eating a good helping of leafy vegetables a day can lower the risk of developing colo-rectal cancer by 46 per cent. Some vegetables have also been linked to lower incidence of colon cancer – they are vegetables of the cruciferous family such as cabbage, cauliflower, broccoli, Pak choi, Brussels sprouts, etc, but spinach, lettuce, tomatoes, orange juice, carrots, celery also have a preventative action.

Population and dietary studies showed that men who eat oily fish or took a fish oil supplement had reduced levels of colon cancer.

Yoghurt may protect against colon cancer. Lactobacillus acidophilus slows down development of colonic tumours and yoghurt eaters have a lower than average incidence of this sort of cancer.

Researchers have put forward the theory that eating olive oil may have a preventative effect on the development of colon cancer.

Taking a selenium supplement seems to lower the risk. Exercise also appears to have a preventative effect in colon cancer. Interestingly, the oral contraceptive pill has been shown to have a protective effect.

High levels of calcium may also prevent colon cancer. Taking a supplement of 1200-1900mg per day reduced the incidence of cancer by 75 per cent.

Prostate cancer

This is now the second most common cancer in UK men, at 21,000 cases per year. It is the seventh most common cause of cancer deaths, killing about 10,000 men per year (three to four per cent of male deaths). Cases of prostate cancer have doubled in the last 20 years in the under 60s – the survival rate is 50 per cent.

Research has suggested a dietary link between prostate cancer and saturated fats. A recent study in Seattle, USA, suggested that a high intake of vegetables, particularly cruciferous, was associated with a reduced risk of cancer of the prostate gland. Interestingly, in parts of Asia where there is a high intake of soya products, prostate cancer levels are low. Phyto-oestrogens and lignans, natural chemicals contained in these products, seem likely to play a part in preventing many cancers that are hormone-dependent.

Controversially, it has been suggested that lower levels of prostate cancer may be due to higher than average exposure to sunlight.

Lycopene, found as the natural red colour in tomatoes and melons, protects against development of prostate cancer – a high intake of tomato products has been associated with a decreased risk. Lycopene is now available as a supplement in health shops. Research shows that a group of men treated with this supplement showed signs that their tumours had shrunk and become less malignant. Lycopene may also play a part in prevention.

Several studies show that regular consumption of fat, particularly saturated fat, (red meat, milk and dairy products) is associated with an increased risk of prostate cancer. A recently published American study from Harvard University looked at the eating habits of 21,000 American doctors over 11 years. They found that 1100 of them developed prostate cancer – they were the people who consumed the most dairy produce.

Bladder cancer

Bladder cancer affects 12,500 men and women per year, seven out of 10 are men – survival rate is 66 per cent. Risk factors include smoking and certain industrial chemicals.

This cancer occurs most commonly in men aged between 50-70 years. It is more frequent in those who drink alcohol and cola drinks and in smokers. It has been known for many years that 500mg of vitamin C three times a day can prevent recurrence with no significant unwanted effects.

Testicular cancer

This is the most common cancer in young men aged 15-49 (affecting 1600 every year). Fortunately, 90 per cent make a full recovery and survival, if the tumour is caught early, is almost 100 per cent. Testicular cancer is associated with undescended testicles, but there may be a risk in men whose diets are high in red meat and milk or low in fruits and vegetables.

Stomach cancer

Stomach cancer affects 10,500 people per year. Epidemiological studies have noted that there is a high incidence of stomach cancers in populations who eat large amounts of smoked foods and those who do a lot of barbecuing. It is thought that the burnt fat irritates the stomach lining leading to cancer of the stomach. A high fruit intake may give a protective effect as can cruciferous vegetables (see above). Two tablespoonfuls of cooked cabbage daily have also been found to help prevent stomach cancer. People who eat the most garlic have lower levels of stomach cancer.

Liver cancer

This is the sixth most common cancer in the world. Patients who have hepatitis B or C, which is due to a viral infection, have a greater risk than unaffected people of developing liver cancer.

Ingesting aflatoxins – a result of mould contamination of grains or nuts – can also cause liver cancer. Being both affected with hepatitis and exposed to aflatoxin increases the risk of contracting liver cancer considerably.

Skin cancer

This cancer is increasing, possibly due to more exposure to sunlight. The chemicals in cosmetics and foaming agents in soaps must not be ignored as possible causative agents as many tumours develop on skin surfaces not usually exposed to sunlight. Fruit and vegetables help to prevent skin cancer when taken with a low fat diet .

What is a portion of fruit and vegetables?

Many people are unsure what amounts to a portion of fruit and vegetables. This comprises:

- One apple, pear, banana, or other piece of fruit; two to three smaller fruits such as kiwi fruit or Sharon fruit; two to three tablespoonfuls of strawberries, grapes or raspberries or other soft fruit; a quarter of a pint of fruit juice; one slice of melon or pineapple or half a grapefruit.

- Two tablespoonfuls of peas, cabbage, broccoli, beetroot, spinach, carrots, parsnips, or courgettes.

- Three tablespoonfuls of beans such as pinto, haricot, lima, runner, French, or sweet corn.

- One dessert bowl of salad vegetables.

19 | References

ABPI Data sheet compendium 2000-2001.

Brinker F, "Herb and drug interactions" 2nd Edition, Eclectic Medical Publications 1998.

British Herbal Pharmacopoeia 1983, British Herbal Medicine Association 1983

Castleman M, "Healing herbs: The ultimate guide to the curative power of nature's medicines" Rodale Press 1991

Clinical evidence, BMJ Publication June 2001

Dukes JA, "The Green Pharmacy" Rodale Press 1997

Newman C, Anderson L, Phillipson DJ, "Herbal medicines: A Guide for Health Care professionals" The Pharmaceutical Press, London 1996.

Mills SY, "The A-Z of Modern Herbalism" Paragon 1993

Mowrey DB, "The scientific validation of herbal medicine" New Canaan CT Keats Publishing 1986

PDR for herbal medicines, Medical Economics Co 2000.

OTHER BOOKS from AMBERWOOD PUBLISHING:

AROMATHERAPY
Aromatherapy – A Guide for Home Use by Christine Westwood. £1.99.
Aromatherapy – For Stress Management by Christine Westwood. £3.50.
Aromatherapy – For Healthy Legs and Feet by Christine Westwood. £2.99.
Aromatherapy – A Nurses Guide by Ann Percival. £2.99.
Aromatherapy – A Nurses Guide for Women by Ann Percival. £2.99.
Aromatherapy – Simply For You by Marion Del Gaudio Mak. £2.99.
Aroma Science – The Chemistry & Bioactivity of Essential Oils by Dr Maria Lis-Balchin. £5.99.
Aromatherapy – Essential Oils in Colour by Dr. Rosemary Caddy. £9.99.
Aromatherapy – The Essential Blending Guide by Dr. Rosemary Caddy. £12.99
Aromatherapy Lexicon – The Essential Reference by Geoff Lyth and Sue Charles. £4.99.
Aromatherapy – The Baby Book by Marion Del Gaudio Mak. £3.99
Aromatherapy – The Pregnancy Book by Jennie Supper. £5.99

HERBAL
Ginkgo Biloba – Ancient Medicine by Dr Desmond Corrigan. £2.99.
Echinacea – Indian Medicine for the Immune System by Dr Desmond Corrigan. £2.99.
Herbal Medicine for Sleep & Relaxation by Dr Desmond Corrigan. £2.99.
Garlic– How Garlic Protects Your Heart by Prof E. Ernst. £3.99.
Phytotherapy – Fifty Vital Herbs by Andrew Chevallier. £6.99
Natural Taste – Herbal Teas, A Guide for Home Use by Andrew Chevallier. £3.50.
Woman Medicine – Vitex Agnus Castus by Simon Mills. £2.99.
Menopause – The Herbal Way by Andrew Chevallier. £5.99
Herbal First Aid – Natural Medicine by Andrew Chevallier. £3.50.
Plant Medicine – A Guide for Home Use by Charlotte Mitchell. £2.99.

GENERAL HEALTHCARE
Insomnia – Doctor I Can't Sleep by Dr Adrian Williams. £2.99.
Eyecare Eyewear – For Better Vision by Mark Rossi. £3.99.
Arthritis and Rheumatism – The Sufferers Guide by Dr John Cosh. £4.95.
Feng Shui – A Guide for Home Use by Karen Ward. £2.99

NUTRITION
Causes & Prevention of Vitamin Deficiency by Dr L. Mervyn. £2.99
Vitamins ABC and Other Food Facts (for Children) by E. Palmer. £3.99
All You Ever Wanted To Know About Vitamins by Dr Leonard Mervyn. £6.99.

CALL FOR INFORMATION: **(01634) 290115**

6. Replace "I can't" with "I can" and "I will."

7. Treat yourself generously, the way you want others to treat you.

8. Be compassionate. Love yourself and others will love you.

9. Remember that you are an individual expression of God. As a work of God's art, you are priceless and irreplaceable.

10. Visualize what you want from life, then work toward it. See it, then be it.

11. Allow time to be by yourself, with yourself. Take time to appreciate yourself.

12. Enjoy your uniqueness. Out of all the billions of people since the beginning of time, there has never been, and never will be, another you.

13. Realize that you are important to the entire world; what happens to the world begins with you.

About Wally Amos

Today, his name is a household word. Wally's most recent venture is Chip and Cookie, LLC, a retail store in Hawaii and online at www.chipandcookie.com, a business featuring two chocolate-chip cookie plush character dolls, Chip & Cookie, created by Christine Harris-Amos. In 1992, he formed Uncle Wally's Muffin Company, which produces a full line of muffins. As founder of Famous Amos Cookies in 1975 and the father of the gourmet chocolate-chip cookie industry, he has used his fame to support many educational causes. Wally was National Spokesman for Literacy Volunteers of America from 1979 until 2002, when they merged with Laubach Literacy Council to create ProLiteracy Worldwide. He now refers to himself as a literacy advocate whose primary focus is creating awareness of the values and benefits of reading aloud to children. He is also a board member of the National Center for Family Literacy and Communities in Schools.

Wally Amos has been the recipient of many honors and awards. He gave the shirt off his back and his battered Panama hat to the Smithsonian Institution's Warshaw Collection of Business Americana. He has been inducted into the Babson College Academy of Distinguished Entrepreneurs, and has received the Horatio Alger Award, The President's Award for Entrepreneurial Excellence, and The National Literacy Leadership Award.

In addition to this book, Wally has authored many other books, including his autobiography, *The Famous Amos Story: The Face That Launched a Thousand Chips, The Power of Self-Esteem*, and *Be Positive! Be Positive!*

Over the years, Wally Amos has acted in a number of network sitcoms and appeared on hundreds of interview shows, news programs, educational programs, and commercials. On the lecture circuit, he addresses audiences at corporations, industry associations, and universities with his inspiring "do it" philosophy. His fame is grounded in quality, substance, and a positive attitude.